Head and Neck Cancers

Editor

RATHAN M. SUBRAMANIAM

PET CLINICS

www.pet.theclinics.com

Consulting Editor
ABASS ALAVI

April 2022 • Volume 17 • Number 2

ELSEVIER

1600 John F. Kennedy Boulevard • Suite 1800 • Philadelphia, Pennsylvania, 19103-2899

http://www.pet.theclinics.com

PET CLINICS Volume 17, Number 2
April 2022 ISSN 1556-8598, ISBN-13: 978-0-323-84938-8

Editor: John Vassallo (j.vassallo@elsevier.com)
Developmental Editor: Karen Solomon

PET Clinics (ISSN 1556-8598) is published quarterly by Elsevier Inc., 360 Park Avenue South, New York, NY 10010-1710. Months of issue are January, April, July, and October. Periodicals postage paid at New York, NY, and additional mailing offices. Subscription prices per year are $262.00 (US individuals), $526.00 (US institutions), $100.00 (US students), $290.00 (Canadian individuals), $552.00 (Canadian institutions), $100.00 (Canadian students), $283.00 (foreign individuals), $552.00 (foreign institutions), and $140.00 (foreign students). To receive student and resident rate, orders must be accompanied by name of affiliated institution, date of term, and the signature of program/residency coordinator on institution letterhead. Orders will be billed at individual rate until proof of status is received. Foreign air speed delivery is included in all Clinics subscription prices. All prices are subject to change without notice. POSTMASTER: Send address changes to PET Clinics, Elsevier Health Sciences Division, Subscription Customer Service, 3251 Riverport Lane, Maryland Heights, MO 63043. **Customer Service: 1-800-654-2452 (U.S. and Canada); 314-447-8871 (outside U.S. and Canada). Fax: 314-447-8029. E-mail: journalscustomerservice-usa@elsevier.com (for print support); journalsonlinesupport-usa@elsevier.com (for online support).**

Reprints. For copies of 100 or more of articles in this publication, please contact the Commercial Reprints Department, Elsevier Inc., 360 Park Avenue South, New York, NY 10010-1710. Tel.: 212-633-3874; Fax: 212-633-3820; E-mail: reprints@elsevier.com.

PET Clinics is covered in MEDLINE/PubMed (Index Medicus).

Contributors

CONSULTING EDITOR

ABASS ALAVI, MD, MD (Hon), PhD (Hon), DSc (Hon)
Professor of Radiology and Neurology,
Director of Research Education, Division of
Nuclear Medicine, Department of Radiology,
Hospital of the University of Pennsylvania,
University of Pennsylvania Perelman School of
Medicine, Philadelphia, Pennsylvania, USA

EDITOR

RATHAN M. SUBRAMANIAM, MD, PhD, MPH, MBA
Professor of Radiology and Nuclear Medicine,
Dean's Office, Otago Medical School,
University of Otago, Dunedin, New Zealand;
Department of Radiology, Duke University,
Durham, North California, USA

AUTHORS

ABDELRAHMAN SHERIF ABDALLA, MD
Division of Oncology, Department of Medicine,
Stanford Cancer Institute, Stanford, California,
USA

CHANDRASEKHAR BAL, MD, DNB, DSc, FAMS, FNASc, FASc
Professor and Head, Department of Nuclear
Medicine, AIIMS, New Delhi, India

STEPHEN M. BROSKI, MD
Department of Radiology, Mayo Clinic,
Rochester, Minnesota, USA

DHRITIMAN CHAKRABORTY, MD, DM
Assistant Professor, Department of Nuclear
and Experimental Medical Sciences, Institute
of Post Graduate Medical Education and
Research/SSKM Hospital, Kolkata, West
Bengal, India

SALMAN ERAJ, MD
Department of Radiation Oncology, The
University of Texas Southwestern Medical
Center, Dallas, Texas, USA

CHRISTOPHER H. HUNT, MD
Departments of Radiology and Neurology,
Mayo Clinic, Rochester, Minnesota, USA

DEREK R. JOHNSON, MD
Departments of Radiology and Neurology,
Mayo Clinic, Rochester, Minnesota, USA

ASHA KANDATHIL, MD
Department of Radiology, The University of
Texas Southwestern Medical Center, Dallas,
Texas, USA

DIKHRA KHAN, MD
Senior Resident, Department of Nuclear
Medicine, AIIMS, New Delhi, India

SAAD A. KHAN, MD
Division of Oncology, Department of Medicine, Stanford Cancer Institute, Stanford, California, USA

CHARLES MARCUS, MD
Division of Nuclear Medicine and Molecular Imaging, Department of Radiology and Imaging Services, Emory University Hospital, Atlanta, Georgia, USA

ANNIE T. PACKARD, MD
Department of Radiology, Mayo Clinic, Rochester, Minnesota, USA

SARA SHEIKHBAHAEI, MD, MPH
The Russell H. Morgan Department of Radiology and Radiological Science, Johns Hopkins Medical Institutions, Baltimore, Maryland, USA

DAVID J. SHER, MD, MPH
Department of Radiation Oncology, The University of Texas Southwestern Medical Center, Dallas, Texas, USA

NATASHA D. SHEYBANI, PhD
Division of Oncology, Department of Medicine, Stanford Cancer Institute, Stanford, California, USA; Department of Biomedical Engineering, University of Virginia, Charlottesville, Virginia, USA

LILJA B. SOLNES, MD, MBA
The Russell H. Morgan Department of Radiology and Radiological Science, Johns Hopkins Medical Institutions, Baltimore, Maryland, USA

RATHAN M. SUBRAMANIAM, MD, PhD, MPH, MBA
Professor of Radiology and Nuclear Medicine, Dean's Office, Otago Medical School, University of Otago, Dunedin, New Zealand; Department of Radiology, Duke University, Durham, North California, USA

VARUT VARDHANABHUTI, MBBS, FRCR, PhD
Clinical Assistant Professor, Department of Diagnostic Radiology, Li Ka Shing Faculty of Medicine, University of Hong Kong, Hong Kong SAR, China

CHENYI XIE, MBBS
Department of Diagnostic Radiology, Li Ka Shing Faculty of Medicine, University of Hong Kong, Hong Kong SAR, China

HELENA YOU, MD
Department of Radiology, Stanford University School of Medicine, Stanford, California, USA

Contents

Preface: Head and Neck Cancer and PET/Computed Tomography   xi

Rathan M. Subramaniam

Clinical Role of Positron Emission Tomography/Computed Tomography Imaging in Head and Neck Squamous Cell Carcinoma   213

Abdelrahman Sherif Abdalla, Natasha D. Sheybani, and Saad A. Khan

Head and neck squamous cell carcinoma (HNSCC) imaging is nearly synonymous with positron emission tomography (PET) scans. Many of the nearly 60,000 newly diagnosed patients with HNSCC in the US—and 900,000 worldwide—will undergo a PET scan, if not multiple, throughout the course of their care. In this review, we describe the clinical utility of PET scans in HNSCC, emphasizing whereby their input is most impactful in improving patient outcomes as well as scenarios whereby PET/CT scans should be avoided. We also describe important considerations for capturing and processing PET scans with a special focus on the important role of tumor volume segmentation, scan timing relative to therapy, and concurrent conditions (eg, COVID-19). In addition, we will illustrate the latest innovations in the management of HNSCC. This article also will delve to exhibit novel potential biomarkers in the management of HNSCC. Finally, we describe future directions for PET imaging, including the advent of novel PET radiotracers as an alternative to 18F-fluorodeoxyglucose (18F-FDG).

PET Imaging of Oral Cavity and Oropharyngeal Cancers   223

Charles Marcus and Rathan M. Subramaniam

Fluorine-18 fluorodeoxyglucose PET/computed tomography (^{18}F-FDG PET/CT) plays an important role in the staging, treatment planning, treatment response assessment, detecting recurrent disease, and predicting prognosis in patients with oral cavity and oropharyngeal squamous cell carcinoma. PET/CT has advantage especially in the detection of nodal, distant metastatic disease and second primary malignancy. PET/MR provides superior soft tissue contrast while decreasing radiation exposure, which is advantageous in evaluation of the primary tumor.

PET/Computed Tomography: Laryngeal and Hypopharyngeal Cancers   235

Asha Kandathil and Rathan M. Subramaniam

Treatment of laryngeal and hypopharyngeal tumors with surgery, radiation therapy, and chemotherapy is aimed at improving survival and preserving function. PET with fluorodeoxyglucose F 18 (^{18}F FDG-PET)/computed tomography is the standard of care and an integral part of staging and treatment response assessment in patients with laryngeal and hypopharyngeal cancers. Knowledge of cross-sectional laryngeal and hypopharyngeal anatomy, expected patterns of tumor spread, and awareness of physiologic FDG uptake in head and neck structures is essential for accurate TNM staging. ^{18}F FDG-PET/computed tomography is superior to anatomic imaging in identifying posttreatment local, regional, and distant tumor recurrence.

18F-fluorodeoxyglucose PET/Computed Tomography: Head and Neck Salivary Gland Tumors   **249**

Stephen M. Broski, Derek R. Johnson, Annie T. Packard, and Christopher H. Hunt

Salivary gland tumors (SGTs) are a heterogeneous group of neoplasms arising from the 3 pairs of major salivary glands (parotid, submandibular, and sublingual) or numerous minor salivary glands located throughout the oral cavity. This review discusses the role of PET/computed tomography (CT) in evaluation of SGTs, including staging, restaging, prognostication, and response assessment. 18F-fluorodeoxyglucose (FDG) PET/CT is useful for staging and restaging malignant SGTs and offers important prognostic information in these patients. It is less useful for differentiating benign and malignant SGTs. Non-FDG PET radiotracers, perineural spread, parotid incidentalomas, and interpretative pitfalls are discussed as well.

Positron Emission Tomography/Computed Tomography in Thyroid Cancer   **265**

Chandrasekhar Bal, Dhritiman Chakraborty, and Dikhra Khan

Fluorine-18-fluorodeoxyglucose-positron emission tomography/computed tomography (18F-FDG PET/CT) plays an important role in the management of thyroid malignancies. Incidentally found FDG avid nodule needs further workup to rule out its malignant potential. 18F-FDG PET/CT has a proven role in detecting recurrent disease or the metastatic workup of the thyroglobulin elevated negative radioiodine scan (TENIS) scenario. In managing histologically aggressive carcinoma of the thyroid, 18F-FDG PET/CT has a proven role. The theranostic potential has been explored with PET/CT using 68Ga-SSA, 68Ga-PSMA,68Ga-FAPI, and 68Ga-DOTA-RGD. The 124I PET/CT role is just being investigated for better spatial resolution and helps in dosimetry.

PET/CT: Nasopharyngeal Cancers   **285**

Chenyi Xie and Varut Vardhanabhuti

PET/CT scan has been used as a tool for the diagnosis and management of nasopharyngeal carcinoma (NPC). It has been proven to be highly valuable for the imaging and management of patients with NPC with strengths in N and M staging as well as treatment planning and is recommended to be incorporated into the standard clinical assessment. Novel quantitative techniques such as the use of radiomics may provide valuable prognostic information.

PET/CT: Radiation Therapy Planning in Head and Neck Cancer   **297**

Salman Eraj and David J. Sher

Fluorine-18-fluorodeoxyglucose (FDG) positron emission tomography (PET) has an integral role in modern radiotherapy planning for most patients with head and neck malignancies. Fluorine-18-fluorodeoxyglucose-positron emission tomography/computed tomography (FDG-PET/CT) should guide standard target delineation and has emerging roles in dose and volume modification for escalation/de-escalation and adaptive radiotherapy. This article discusses the integration of PET/CT into radiotherapy planning.

2-Deoxy-2-[^{18}F] Fluoro-D-Glucose PET/Computed Tomography: Therapy Response Assessment in Head and Neck Cancer   307

Sara Sheikhbahaei, Rathan M. Subramaniam, and Lilja B. Solnes

^{18}F-FDG-PET/CT (2-deoxy-2-[^{18}F] fluoro-D-glucose PET/computed tomography) is a reliable modality for accurate assessment of treatment response, early detection of recurrence, or second primary tumors in head and neck squamous cell carcinoma (HNSCC), if performed at the appropriate time after therapy. This review focuses on the utility of posttreatment ^{18}F-FDG-PET/CT in HNSCC, reviews the expected imaging findings and pitfalls after treatments, summarizes common ^{18}F-FDG-based quantitative and qualitative response assessment methods, and discusses the value of imaging surveillance in HNSCC. We also provide an overview of recently approved immune checkpoint inhibitors in HNSCC and current recommendations on immunotherapy-response monitoring.

PET/Computed Tomography: Post-therapy Follow-up in Head and Neck Cancer   319

Helena You and Rathan M. Subramaniam

PET/computed tomography (CT) is a valuable tool in post-therapy follow-up of head and neck cancers. PET/CT is sensitive and specific, can detect recurrences that otherwise may be missed on routine clinical examination or conventional imaging, and also can have an impact on patient management. National Comprehensive Cancer Network guidelines recommend PET/CT be performed within 3 months to 6 months after therapy. After this baseline scan, however, further routine PET/CT surveillance in asymptomatic patients has unclear benefit. Additional post-therapy PET/CT imaging should be individualized to patients based on considerations such as tumor type, stage, prognostic factors, symptoms, and clinical assessment.

PET CLINICS

FORTHCOMING ISSUES

July 2022
FDG vs. non-FDG Tracers in Less Explored Domains: An Appraisal
Sandip Basu, Rakesh Kumar, and Abass Alavi, *Editors*

October 2022
Prostate Cancer
Harshad R. Kulkarni and Abass Alavi, *Editors*

January 2023
Critical Role of PET in Assessing Age Related Disorders
Abass Alavi, Babak Saboury, and Ali Gholamrezanezhad, *Editors*

RECENT ISSUES

January 2022
Artificial Intelligence and PET Imaging, Part II
Babak Saboury, Arman Rahmim, and Eliot Siegel, *Editors*

October 2021
Artificial Intelligence and PET Imaging, Part I
Babak Saboury, Arman Rahmim, and Eliot Siegel, *Editors*

July 2021
Theranostics
Hojjat Ahmadzadehfar and Ali Gholamrezanezhad, *Editors*

THE CLINICS ARE AVAILABLE ONLINE!
Access your subscription at:
www.theclinics.com

PROGRAM OBJECTIVE

The goal of the PET Clinics is to keep practicing radiologists and radiology residents up to date with current clinical practice in positron emission tomography by providing timely articles reviewing the state of the art in patient care.

TARGET AUDIENCE

Practicing radiologists, radiology residents, and other health care professionals who provide patient care utilizing radiologic findings.

LEARNING OBJECTIVES

Upon completion of this activity, participants will be able to:

1. Review the purpose of PET/CT as the standard of care for diagnosing, staging, assessing, and treating head and neck cancers.
2. Discuss the role, response, and benefits of using PET/CT imaging, both traditional and novel, accurately assessing, diagnosing, and treating primary and recurrent head and neck malignancies.
3. Recognize the importance of PET/CT imaging for assessment response, staging, restaging, prognostication, and early detection of recurrence of head and neck malignancies

ACCREDITATION

The Elsevier Office of Continuing Medical Education (EOCME) is accredited by the Accreditation Council for Continuing Medical Education (ACCME) to provide continuing medical education for physicians.

The EOCME designates this journal-based CME activity for a maximum of 9 *AMA PRA Category 1 Credit*(s)™. Physicians should claim only the credit commensurate with the extent of their participation in the activity.

All other health care professionals requesting continuing education credit for this enduring material will be issued a certificate of participation.

DISCLOSURE OF CONFLICTS OF INTEREST

The EOCME assesses conflict of interest with its instructors, faculty, planners, and other individuals who are in a position to control the content of CME activities. All relevant conflicts of interest that are identified are thoroughly vetted by EOCME for fair balance, scientific objectivity, and patient care recommendations. EOCME is committed to providing its learners with CME activities that promote improvements or quality in healthcare and not a specific proprietary business or a commercial interest.

The planning committee, staff, authors, and editors listed below have identified no financial relationships or relationships to products or devices they or their spouse/life partner have with commercial interest related to the content of this CME activity:

Abdelrahman Sherif Abdalla, MD; Chandrasekhar Bal, MD, DNB, DSc, FAMS, FNASc, FASc; Stephen M. Broski, MD; Dhritiman Chakraborty, MD, DM; Salman Eraj, MD; Christopher H. Hunt, MD; Derek R. Johnson, MD; Asha Kandathil, MD; Saad A. Khan, MD; Dikhra Khan, MD; Charles Marcus, MD; Annie T. Packard, MD; Sara Sheikhbahaei, MD, MPH; David J. Sher, MD, MPH; Natasha D. Sheybani, PhD; Lilja B. Solnes, MD, MBA; Rathan M. Subramaniam, MD, PhD, MPH, MBA; Doreen Thomas-Payne, MSN, BSN, RN, PMHNP-BC; Varut Vardhanabhuti, MBBS, FRCR, PhD; Mohana Manoj; Chenyi Xie, MBBS; Helena You, MD

UNAPPROVED/OFF-LABEL USE DISCLOSURE

The EOCME requires CME faculty to disclose to the participants:

1. When products or procedures being discussed are off-label, unlabelled, experimental, and/or investigational (not US Food and Drug Administration [FDA] approved); and
2. Any limitations on the information presented, such as data that are preliminary or that represent ongoing research, interim analyses, and/or unsupported opinions. Faculty may discuss information about pharmaceutical agents that is outside of FDA-approved labelling. This information is intended solely for CME and is not intended to promote off-label use of these medications. If you have any questions, contact the medical affairs department of the manufacturer for the most recent prescribing information.

TO ENROLL

To enroll in the PET Clinics Continuing Medical Education program, call customer service at 1-800-654-2452 or sign up online at http://www.theclinics.com/home/cme. The CME program is available to subscribers for an additional annual fee of USD 254.00

METHOD OF PARTICIPATION

In order to claim credit, participants must complete the following:

1. Complete enrolment as indicated above.
2. Read the activity.
3. Complete the CME Test and Evaluation. Participants must achieve a score of 70% on the test. All CME Tests and Evaluations must be completed online.

CME INQUIRIES/SPECIAL NEEDS

For all CME inquiries or special needs, please contact elsevierCME@elsevier.com

Preface

Head and Neck Cancer and PET/Computed Tomography

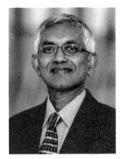

Rathan M. Subramaniam, MD, PhD, MPH, MBA
Editor

Head and Neck Cancer is the seventh most common cancer worldwide and consists of a heterogeneous group of types affecting the upper aerodigestive tract. The most common histologic type is squamous cell cancers, and risk factors include smoking, alcohol, and oncogenic viruses, especially human papilloma virus-16 and -18 (HPV16 & 18) and Epstein-Barr virus for nasopharyngeal cancer. The treatment for head and neck cancers is a multimodal approach with surgery, radiotherapy, chemotherapy, immunotherapy, and other targeted therapies. The prognosis depends on site, stage, and HPV involvement. Five-year survival for patients with stage I to II disease is 70% to 90%, and patients with stage III to IV disease typically have a poorer prognosis. Furthermore, patients with HPV-associated oropharyngeal cancers have an excellent prognosis, approaching 80%, despite the locoregionally advanced disease.

Over the last two decades, it has become a standard clinical practice to obtain an FDG-PET/computed tomography (CT) scan for head and cancer workup, especially for locoregionally advanced disease and identifying distant metastases. FDG-PET/CT is valuable in detecting unknown primary tumors, neck nodal metastases, distant metastases for radiation therapy planning, assessing treatment response, detecting suspected recurrences, and providing a prognosis.

FDG-PET/CT is now widely used in many multi-center clinical trials for diagnosis, staging, and treatment response assessment. For assessment of the primary tumor, a contrast-enhanced CT or MR imaging is essential.

In this issue of *PET Clinics*, leading international authors discuss the value of PET/CT in head and neck cancers, including oropharynx, larynx, nasopharynx, thyroid cancers; salivary gland tumors; neck nodal assessment; radiation therapy planning; therapy assessment; and follow-up. In addition, novel diagnostic tests, such as salivary and serum markers, novel FDG-PET image analysis, novel PET radiopharmaceuticals, and evolving therapies, such as immunotherapy, are discussed. We hope you find this fine collection of articles valuable for your clinical practice and advancing knowledge. These articles synthesize the evolution of FDG-PET/CT over the last two decades, and its value for head and neck cancer management and contribution to the field.

Rathan M. Subramaniam, MD, PhD, MPH, MBA
Dean's Office
Otago Medical School
University of Otago
Dunedin 9016, New Zealand

E-mail address:
rathan.subramaniam@otago.ac.nz

PET Clin 17 (2022) xi
https://doi.org/10.1016/j.cpet.2022.02.005
1556-8598/22/© 2022 Published by Elsevier Inc.

Preface

Head and Neck Cancer and PET/Computed Tomography

Clinical Role of Positron Emission Tomography/ Computed Tomography Imaging in Head and Neck Squamous Cell Carcinoma

Abdelrahman Sherif Abdalla, MD[a,1], Natasha D. Sheybani, PhD[a,b,1], Saad A. Khan, MD[a,*]

KEYWORDS

- Head and neck cancer • iPET • Head and neck squamous cell carcinoma • COVID-19

KEY POINTS

- The modern clinical practice of head and neck oncology nearly mandates PET/CT be performed on patients at the time of diagnosis, treatment decision-making, and surveillance of HNSCC.
- PET/CT is clearly beneficial in occult primary, advanced disease, and 12 week response assessment after definitive chemotherapy and radiation.
- Advances in nuclear medicine are reducing the horrific personal and public health burden of this disease and minimizing the side effects of our intensive treatments.

BACKGROUND

Every year, head and neck squamous cell carcinoma (HNSCC) affects more than 66,000 people in the US and 900,000 worldwide.[1,2] This number only partially represents each individual tragedy of pain, death, and long-term disability that each individual case represents. HNSCC is a tremendous health burden that in many cases is preventable, and the amount of suffering can be substantially reduced by delivering the best standard of care to our patients in terms of work-up, imaging and treatment selection to all patients.[3] HNSCC demonstrates a skewed gender distribution complicated by treatment and outcome disparity by gender.[3] While men occupying the

highest numerical portion of those affected,[1,2] a study reported worse outcomes and undertreatment for women when compared to men.[4] Improving outcomes for all these patients may be achieved by reviewing the integral role of nuclear medicine imaging in this disease, and it is our goal in writing this article.

Surgical and radiation treatment modalities for cancers that arise in the head and neck region require detailed mapping of areas of suspected disease involvement and their spatial relation to critical anatomic structures such as nerves, vessels, and muscles.[5] In this review we will focus primarily on more than 90% of head and neck cancers which are comprised by the squamous cell carcinoma subtype. However, for clinicians,

COI information: The authors do not have any conflicts of interest to report.

[a] Division of Oncology, Department of Medicine, Stanford Cancer Institute, 875 Blake Wilbur Avenue, Stanford, CA 94304, USA; [b] Division of Oncology, Department of Medicine, Stanford Cancer Institute, 875 Blake Wilbur Avenue, Stanford, CA 94304, USA
[1] Authors contributed equally.
* Corresponding author. Division of Oncology, Department of Medicine, Stanford Cancer Institute, 875 Blake Wilbur Avenue Stanford, CA 94304.
E-mail address: Saad.A.Khan@Stanford.edu

it is clear that even the term "HNSCC" is an over-simplification that encompasses multiple entirely distinct diseases that are often considered together under a unitary diagnostic misnomer.[6] An analysis of head and neck cancers found 18 distinct ICD-10 code headings, and researchers involved with SEER-Medicare are aware that "head and neck cancer" data are spread across 3 separate data files.[7–9] Laryngeal and oropharyngeal squamous cancers differ markedly in etiology, treatment approach, and survival outcomes. HNSCC is unique in that the anatomic relation of primary cancer can occasionally be determined with high precision under direct visualization. However, in modern treatment settings, it is essential not to just visually determine the areas that are involved but also the relation of these areas to delicate structures such as underlying critical structures. Radiation treatment and organ-sparing surgeries have yielded noteworthy improvements in patient survival rates and quality of life. Yet, highly intensive treatment of head and neck cancers—including radiation, surgery, and chemotherapy—can result in significant morbidities including high rates of mucositis, xerostomia, dysphagia, and permanent damage to vital physiologic organs such as eyes, tongue, and vocal cords.[10]

In this clinically oriented review, we highlight the role of the latest innovations in positron emission tomography (PET) and computed tomography (CT) imaging for the management of HNSCC. We discuss the impact of PET/CT on diagnosis, treatment selection, and surveillance. Finally, we discuss future roles for PET/CT in the management of HNSCC in particular and, in selected other rare cancers that arise in the head and neck region.

Overview of Positron Emission Tomography/ Computed Tomography in Head and Neck Cancer

HNSCC diagnosis is a dynamic process whereby clinical, laboratory, and radiographic data must be rapidly incorporated into the best objective description of the patient's disease state. In recent years, the diagnostic process has been standardized by the publication of national guidelines, because a proper work-up is essential for optimal treatment selection. Histopathological confirmation of HNSCC triggers the need for the accurate staging of head and neck cancer. This is initially performed by physical examination and imaging by MR imaging which is often the preferred method for assessing the primary site of disease and other sites of abnormality. Thoughtful,

evidence-based incorporation of CT or PET/CT in some cases is essential for the accurate localization of primary tumor and to determine its extent, for assessing nodal involvement, and for determining the presence or absence of metastasis.[11]

PET/CT uniquely supplements the diagnostic process by detecting nodal involvement and distant metastases with high metabolic activity. This is especially important in anatomically normal-appearing areas whereby the malignancy may be obscured by surrounding nonmalignant tissue, or when a tumor is present in an area that is not enlarged by size criteria. An example of the staging of oropharyngeal cancer as one type of head neck cancer demonstrates how clinicians evaluate the primary site, nodal involvement (by both size and number criteria), and the presence of distant disease. Accurate tumor, node, and metastasis (TNM) staging is essential to avoid over-treating or under-treating cancers or regions, and minor variations of these staging values can dramatically change the expected prognosis and our therapeutic recommendations.

PATIENT PERSPECTIVE OF POSITRON EMISSION TOMOGRAPHY SCANS

The oncology literature often discusses the utility and performance of PET/CT in highly technical terms. However, for clinicians and nuclear medicine specialists alike, it is helpful to remember that each PET/CT we view is likely to represent a major turning point in our patients' lives. Whether it is a new diagnosis of cancer, news of cure, or recurrence each scan will be remembered by the patient long after we have moved on. In cancer center clinic rooms, because of its easily understood vivid colors PET/CT is commonly presented to the patient and their families as evidence of resounding success or to highlight areas of concern. These computer screens demonstrating "before" and "after" cancer treatment images are often photographed by patients and shared in celebration with friends and family members.

Patients believe that the "best" HNSCC imaging modality is a PET/CT and will regularly ask why it is not ordered, even though studies suggest that PET/CT scan anxiety is significant.[12] Our approach to patients is to describe nuclear medicine imaging such as PET/CT as one tool out of many to help us arrive at the most accurate description of the extent of cancer, and which is used when necessary. The nuclear medicine specialist helps the clinician gain the best description of reality and patients do recognize the entire team's tremendous contributions to their cure and longevity.

CURRENT STANDARDS OF CARE IN HEAD AND NECK CANCER MANAGEMENT

Understanding the role of nuclear medicine imaging in HNSCC requires a brief introduction of common treatments and the oncologists involved. Most patients who develop abnormalities in the head and neck present to an otolaryngologist or head and neck surgeon initially. As head and neck tumors are often visible or palpable most tumors are identified early and are treated by a surgeon without the involvement of other cancer specialists.

Management depends on the stage and subtype of HNSCC due to the complex nature and the high potential for metastases. Depending on the HNSCC stage, management involves either surgery alone or the combination of surgery and radiation. Indeed, latest advances in surgery allowed for minimally invasive surgical procedures as transoral robotic surgery (TORS) and transoral laser microsurgery (TLM) which significantly reduced postoperative complications including pain management and reduced the overall expenses of cancer treatment.

- Locally confined cancer with single nodal involvement can be managed with a single therapeutic modality (surgery or radiation) with approximately 90% 3-year survival.[13]
- More Advanced tumors require interventions guided by pathologic risk factors and include postsurgical radiation, chemotherapy, or chemoradiation.[14,15]

While the need for nuclear medicine imaging in locally advanced and clinically node involving cases is clear, there are high-level evidence, suggesting the use of PET/CT in smaller volume disease may be of value. In the prospective clinical trial ACRIN 6685, there was superiority of PET/CT in not only optimal workup but also altering treatment decisions. That study showed a negative predictive value (NPV) of 0.94 for FDG PET/CT in cN0 HNSCC and overall changed the surgical plan in 22% of patients.

PATHOLOGY AND IMMUNE LANDSCAPE OF HEAD AND NECK CANCER
Pathology

The large majority of head and neck cancers are of squamous histology, with other histologies such as melanoma, lymphoma, neuroendocrine tumors (NETs), adenocarcinomas and undifferentiated tumors making up the bulk of the remainder.[16,17] Cancers of the thyroid gland arise in the head and neck region but the vast majority are treated surgically and never have a PET/CT performed.

Even within HNSCC, there are wide variations in pathologic descriptions of clinical significance. More recently HPV status or expression of the p16 protein has become imperative to report in oropharyngeal cancer specimens, as that affects diagnosis, staging, and clinical trial eligibility. HPV viral onco-proteins, E6 and E7, cause the degradation of, p53 and pRb, which are the main tumor suppressor proteins leading to tumorigenesis and persistent infection leads to constant expression of E6 and E7 which is required for tumor maintenance.[18,19]

Positron Emission Tomography/Computed Tomography Relation to Head and Neck Squamous Cell Carcinoma Pathology

Head and neck tumors represent a diverse spectrum of biological growths with a varying affinity for FDG. Many high-grade malignancies such as HNSCC, aggressive lymphomas, and radioiodine refractory thyroid cancers are highly metabolically active and thus tend to be well-visualized on these PET/CTs. Other cancers that have less cell turnover or unique biology such as well-differentiated thyroid cancers or NETs may either not be visualized on PET/CT or may require alternate radiotracers.

Though rates of PET/CT usage across the various histologies are not reported, head and neck cancer experienced clinicians will often supplement their workup of head and neck tumors with nuclear medicine imaging. In even relatively slow-growing tumors such as esthesioneuroblastoma, a retrospective analysis of 28 patients at a single center who underwent 77 FDG PET/CT found a median SUVmax of 8.68 (range 3.6–23.3) at the primary tumor site and 8.57 (range 1.9–27.2) at metastatic sites, resulting in the upstaging of 36% of patients.[20] Across all varying histologies including within HNSCC, FDG PET/CT imaging that reveals higher metabolic activity/SUV readings during the initial workup may raise clinical suspicion that these tumors are more aggressive. In clinical practice, higher metabolic activity on PET/CT does not automatically signify a worse outcome or trigger more aggressive treatments.

TYPICAL USE FLUORINE-18-FLUORODEOXYGLUCOSE-POSITRON EMISSION TOMOGRAPHY/COMPUTED TOMOGRAPHY IMAGING IN HEAD AND NECK CANCER

PET scans using the glucose analog 18F-FDG have become an essential imaging tool for the assessment of HNSCC, especially for accurate staging that reflects potential metastases or second primaries to lungs.[21] The preferential uptake of FDG by malignant cells yields a high tumor-to-background intensity ratio, which provides heightened sensitivity to cancerous tissues. The lengthy scan duration and exposure to radioactivity necessitated by PET imaging remain major drawbacks of using this modality. PET scans are also known to have limited spatial resolution, which hinders the complete visualization of tumor borders and poses challenges for precise contouring. The joint usage of PET and CT scans—as opposed to PET alone—has helped to surmount some of these hurdles, leading to improved identification of tumors and substantially decreased scan times.

The lungs are the most common site of metastasis in HNSCC.[22] In patients with a history of head and neck cancer, new primary lung cancer can occur simultaneously or metachronously, and this is seen in approximately 9% of patients.[22,23] The National Comprehensive Cancer Network (NCCN) recommends that patients with HNSCC undergo PET imaging of the chest at baseline for staging as well as within 6 months following the conclusion of therapy.[24] Routine screening of the abdomen using PET/CT scans is not recommended due to low rates of metastasis to the liver.[25] Often, liver function tests yield abnormal results in patients with HNSCC, but this alone should not be an indication for performing PET/CT scans. Rather, it is recommended that abdominal imaging is performed in a risk-stratified manner as a more cost-effective solution for high-risk groups.[24]

Current Initial Imaging Recommendation in Head and Neck Cancer

18F-FDG PET/CT plays an important role in pretreatment staging, radiotherapy planning, and posttherapy surveillance for head and neck cancers.[26] Cross-sectional modalities such as MR imaging or CT scans are the gold standard for the initial workup of head and neck tumors to localize the primary site of such tumors.[27] Although such modalities can also detect lymph node metastases, they are less accurate than FDG PET/CT scan in detecting locoregional and distant nodal metastases.[28] Therefore, if a primary site cannot be identified on direct visual inspection and MR imaging or CT, then an FDG PET/CT can be used at the point of care. In occult primary HNSCC, cervical lymph nodes are enlarged with no primary site identified in 5% to 10% of head and neck cancer cases, and a PET/CT is performed and can help identify a primary site.[29] The National Comprehensive Cancer Network (NCCN)

recommends using CT scan to assess mediastinal lymph nodes in patients with multi-station nodal involvement, lower neck nodal involvement, or high-grade tumor histology but still recommends using FDG PET/CT scan whenever possible due to the higher sensitivity and specificity.[27] Patients who are undergoing primary surgical management of midline tumors are strongly recommended to undergo FDG PET/CT scan to determine the possibility and the extent of a possible contralateral surgical intervention per NCCN guidelines.[27] The same is true for patients undergoing radiation therapy to determine the nodal involvement with high accuracy.[27]

The addition of PET/CT in this situation would be considered essential, as high rates of sensitivity and specificity have been reported in numerous clinical analyses of occult primary head and neck cancer patients.[26,30,31] Those with more advanced disease such as > T2 primary or locoregional nodal involvement also have a risk of distant metastases. Here the role of PET/CT becomes twofold to further characterize the areas of locoregional involvement as well as to identify any sites of distant metastatic disease. At tertiary medical centers in the US, clinical practice and HNSCC treatment recommendations without PET in these cases would be considered incomplete. Patients that do not undergo a PET/CT include those with early-stage HNSCC whereby a small-sized primary is clearly identified, as the likelihood of nodal involvement is low.

Drawbacks of Fluorine-18-Fluorodeoxyglucose-Positron Emission Tomography/Computed Tomography Scan

Despite its high sensitivity (>95%) for detecting primary head and neck cancers, FDG-PET/CT imaging—particularly when performed with noncontrast enhanced CT—remains limited in its ability to accurately capture how tumors are spreading and interfacing with adjacent structures.[26] To overcome these limitations almost always the nuclear medicine study that is ordered is a contrast-enhanced PET/CT or PET/MR imaging.[32,33] Detection of cervical lymph node involvement has emerged as a major diagnostic role for FDG-PET in the initial diagnosis and prognostication of head and neck cancer. FDG PET shines in terms of detecting head and neck cancer as such modality has both greater sensitivity (86%–100%) and greater specificity (69%–87%) than CT with a sensitivity of 67%–82% and specificity of 25%–56%, for the detection of both primary tumors and lymph node metastases.[34] Also, there are a number of precautions that should be taken into consideration before ordering PET/CT scan to patients. Women patients who are candidates for FDG PET/CT scanning should be screened for pregnancy. Also, patients who are taking metformin for diabetes management should stop metformin the day of the procedure and resume 48 hours postscan in case there is no significant risk for renal dysfunction.[35] Physicians should also take into consideration risk factors for contrast-induced nephropathy including age, chronic kidney injury (CKD), hypertension, and diabetes mellitus and weight risk versus benefits of ordering FDG PET/CT scan for such patients.[36]

Radiation Planning

FDG-PET imaging has been adopted as an important adjunct in radiotherapy planning for head and neck cancer. It offers the ability to delineate gross tumor volumes (GTV) in a more reproducible manner, thereby reducing the likelihood of risk of off-target radiation delivery. Moreover, with the advent of novel PET radiotracers capable of delineating regions of hypoxia or high cellular proliferation in tumors (see *Alternative PET Radiotracers*), radiation planning can be targeted and fine-tuned with the consideration of these characteristics.[37] There is tremendous utility in leveraging PET imaging to aid critical yet basic clinical decisions such as determining GTV, clinical tumor volume and then incorporating all these data to determine the planning treatment volume (PTV). Information from a PET/CT may be used to escalate radiation dose in select subvolumes or otherwise alter the course of treatment. The addition of a radio-sensitizing chemotherapy agent to the radiation is information gathered from a PET scan such as the presence of multiple nodal metastases. Despite the attractive nature of delivering radiation to a PET/CT-defined tumor volume, key limitations have constrained the widespread adoption of this approach. These include finite spatial resolution, false positivity associated with signals from nonmalignant, FDG-avid tissues, and a lack of standardized methodology for the segmentation of target volumes.[38]

Surgery

PET/CT is not routinely performed in patients after they have recently undergone surgery as the procedure itself leads to abnormal metabolic activity that may be completely unrelated to cancer growth. Similarly, successful surgery's goal is to have no metabolically active cancerous tissue remaining, and postsurgical adjuvant therapy is designed to eradicate microscopic disease. Therefore, early PET/CT in this setting is clinically

considered more likely to yield false positives rather than useful information, and PET/CTs are not recommended unless there is some evidence or suspicion of gross disease recurrence.

Surveillance

Surveillance is performed after the conclusion of therapy for head and neck cancer. As primary disease sites treated with radiation or concurrent chemoradiotherapy have seen favorable response rates, the more urgent use case for posttherapy FDG-PET is generally found in the detection of residual disease in lymph nodes of the neck. One benefit in this surveillance setting is that not only can the dimensions of the malignant areas be identified but also changes in metabolic activity can be assessed by comparing to a pretreatment baseline PET/CT scan. However, studies have varied considerably in the timing of response assessment following the conclusion of therapy. For example, while PET scans have been performed as early as 6-weeks postchemoradiotherapy,[39] these can be susceptible to greater false-positive rates by virtue of posttherapy inflammatory changes as well as the protracted timeline on which irradiated cells ultimately die. For this reason, biopsy is often recommended to validate a PET-positive result.[32] In light of these considerations, the emerging consensus holds that PET scans should not be performed any sooner than 10 to 12 weeks after therapy ends.[40,41] While FDG-PET scans are not routinely performed beyond this time frame - unless warranted by areas of concern—studies performing PET at more chronic time points (ie, at 4-months posttreatment and beyond) have seen lower false-positive rates.[42]

NOVEL APPROACHES FOR IMMUNE LANDSCAPE

A major revolution in HNSCC treatment has been the approval of immune checkpoint therapies, either in combination with chemotherapy or as monotherapy.[43–45] The combined positive score (CPS) is a companion diagnostic test that predicts benefit to patients from pembrolizumab usage and is routinely generated by pathologic analysis of the tumor. It is calculated as the percentage of total PD-L1-positive cells (tumor cells, lymphocytes, and macrophages) out of total PD-L1-positive and -negative tumor cells.[46] A CPS of 1 or greater confers on-label usage of pembrolizumab monotherapy,[47] with a putative explanation that the greater the number of immune cells infiltrating the HNSCC equates to greater effector cells that can then destroy the cancer cells after exposure to the anti-PD1 agent. PET/CT using 2-deoxy-2-[fluorine-18] fluoro-D-glucose (18F-FDG) has been proposed as a noninvasive proxy for determining this immune cell infiltration of tumors. However, there are conflicting data about its efficacy and reproducibility. It is not considered standard to use PET/CT imaging to determine the pathologic subtype of cancer or the likelihood of response to immune checkpoint inhibitors.

FUTURE DIRECTIONS AND CONSIDERATIONS

In this review, we have highlighted the central role of PET in the current treatment landscape for HNSCC. Exciting new developments in radiographic technology suggest that PET will take on an even more important role in this disease in the coming years. With an eye toward these future directions, we here highlight areas of research and special considerations relevant to PET usage in head and neck cancers.

Response Assessment (Interim Positron Emission Tomography)

PET/CT is regularly used after the completion of surgery, radiation, and/or systemic therapy treatments to determine if there are any areas of suspicion that need to be addressed immediately or in future imaging plans. Novel use of PET/CT approaches is being considered to escalate or de-escalate treatment, building on experience from other solid cancers. An interim PET (iPET) is regularly performed in diffuse large B cell lymphoma (DLBCL) after the standard cycles of chemotherapy.[48] Qualitative or quantitative comparisons between pretreatment PET/CT findings and those captured after a defined number of initial chemotherapy cycles are used to determine how many additional cycles of chemotherapy patients with DLBCL need to undergo.

A recently introduced criterion for therapy response assessment "Hopkins criteria" sets unified guidelines for interpreting FDG PET/CT scan when assessing the therapeutic response of HNSCC. Such criteria have been validated to have excellent inter-reader agreement and prediction of progression-free survival.[49,50] These criteria are listed later in discussion[49]:

- Response category F-18-FDG uptake at the primary site and nodes less than internal jugular vein (IJV). Complete metabolic response.
- Focal F-18-FDG uptake at the primary site and nodes greater than IJV but less than liver. Likely complete metabolic response.
- Diffuse F-18-FDG uptake at the primary site or nodes is greater than IJV or liver. Likely postradiation inflammation.
- Focal F-18-FDG uptake at the primary site or nodes greater than liver. Likely residual tumor.

- Focal and intense F-18-FDG uptake at the primary site or nodes. Residual tumor.

HNSCC therapy is burdened by significant toxicities, but with better treatments, cancer-related outcomes have improved. There is now a heightened awareness that perhaps the greatest positive impact on patients' lives may come from a gradual de-escalation of treatment. Traditional techniques have used clinical response at the primary HNSCC site to reduce radiation intensity.[51]

Meanwhile, use of an HNSCC iPET has been reported,[13] with a special interest in parameters such as a change between baseline and mid-treatment maximum standardized uptake value (SUVmax) or metabolic tumor volume in a conserved volume of interest; these metrics may be used to determine the likelihood of a given treatment to be effective in cancer control. If these approaches are refined and validated, HNSCC treatments could be escalated or de-escalated for patients on the basis of an iPET. This remains an area whereby prospective clinical trials are clearly needed, as the potential success of such an approach could stand to bear a vast impact on patient lives.[52] HNSCC therapy is burdened by significant toxicities, but with better treatments, cancer-related outcomes have improved. There is now a heightened awareness that perhaps the greatest positive impact on patients' lives may come from a gradual de-escalation of treatment. Traditional techniques have used clinical response at the primary HNSCC site to reduce radiation intensity.[51]

Alternative Positron Emission Tomography Radiotracers

Interpretation of malignancies on PET imaging can be limited by the nonspecific uptake of 18F-FDG by normal or inflammatory tissues. However, recent years have seen the expansion of the capabilities of nuclear medicine in head and neck cancer owing to the advent of more specific radiotracers targeting distinct molecular mechanisms. For example, tumor hypoxia plays an important role in the treatment response of head and neck cancers and commonly underpins radio-resistance. Novel radiotracers enabling in vivo detection of hypoxia include 18F-fluoromisonidazole (18F-FMISO), 18F-fluoroazomycin-arabinofluranoside (18F-FAZA), and 18F-3-[F] fluoro-2-(4-((2-nitro-1H-imidazole-1-yl)methyl)-1H-1,2,3,-triazol-1-yl)-propan-1-ol (18F-HX4). Other radiopharmaceuticals under clinical investigation include 18F-fluorothymidine (18F-FLT), which targets tumor proliferation and the DNA synthetic pathway, as well as 18F-fluoroethyl-L-thyrosine

(18F-FET) and L-(methyl-11C) methionine (11C-MET) for imaging protein synthesis.[26] The role of these non-FDG radiotracers in the PET/CT imaging of head and neck cancers is elsewhere reviewed in greater detail.[53]

Immuno-PET probes have the potential to combine the specificity of monoclonal antibodies with the imaging capabilities of PET to achieve better sensitivity and specificity in detecting primary tumors, nodal involvement, and metastases in the context of head and neck cancer. Zirconium-89-labeled panitumumab is an example of a promising immuno-PET probe that showed preferential tumor uptake corresponding with the expression of HER-1 oncogene.[54] Indeed, the targeted specificity of panitumumab in combination with the quantitative imaging capabilities of PET scan demonstrably led to better detection of micro-metastasis, whereby standard PET imaging methods otherwise fall short. A clinical trial evaluating intravenously delivered panitumumab for metastatic and sentinel lymph node mapping determined 100% sensitivity, 85.8% specificity, and 100% NPV for the detection of occult metastases and 100% accuracy for clinically staging the neck.[55] As such, this modality has the potential to shift the paradigm for sentinel lymph node biopsy by enabling radiotracer injection as a method for the identification of sentinel lymph nodes during surgery.

Finally, to predict response to immunotherapies and contextualize mechanisms of resistance, there is also a growing need for reliable imaging biomarkers of immune response. In an effort to fulfill this need, an 18F-labeled analog of arabino-furanosyl guanine (AraG) has been developed for PET imaging of activated CD8+ T cells. Preliminary findings in 5 patients with head and neck cancer have demonstrated that this tracer is safe and capable of mapping CD8+ T cell biodistribution in both benign and malignant tissues.[56]

COVID-19-Associated Diffuse Lymphadenopathy

The novel coronavirus disease (COVID-19) has given rise to a global pandemic and public health crisis of historic proportions. Recent reports have documented the confounding role that COVID-19 infection and vaccination can play in the interpretation of radiographic imaging of oncology patients. Indeed, patients undergoing FDG-PET/CT imaging after COVID-19 vaccination have seen transient FDG uptake owing to diffuse lymphadenopathy (eg, in axillary, supraclavicular, and cervical lymph nodes) after ipsilateral deltoid vaccination.[57,58] These observations have generated timely and important clinical considerations with respect to the timing of PET/CT imaging relative to COVID-19 vaccination as well as laterality of vaccine injection relative to cancer site.[58]

Head and Neck Neuroendocrine Tumors

Rarely, NETs can arise in the head and neck region, wherein they tend not to take up 18F-FDG. Recent studies have demonstrated the utility of 68Ga-1,4,7,10-tetraazacyclododecane-1,4,7,10-tetraacetic acid (DOTA)–octreotate (68Ga-DOTA-TATE)—a somatostatin analog—for imaging these tumors by the way of cell surface expression of somatostatin receptors. This method is finding clinical utility as a complement to FDG-PET imaging for patient prognosis and management, and has thus become the preferred functional imaging modality for NETs of the head and neck (eg, paragangliomas).[59–61]

THE EVOLVING UTILIZATION OF BIOMARKERS IN HEAD AND NECK SQUAMOUS CELL CARCINOMA

A wide range of new generation of biomarkers has the potential to be used to guide the clinical practice in managing HNSCC.

- Different methylation markers detected in the saliva of patients with HNSCC demonstrated significant correlation to HNSCC and such markers include methylation panel of DAPK1, p16, and RASSF1A genes demonstrated sensitivity of 94% and specificity of 87% which shows potential in screening patients with HNSCC.[62] Also, KIF1A and EDNRB hypermethylation demonstrated 77.4% sensitivity and 93.1% specificity.[62] The combined both panels can achieve high sensitivity and specificity of each marker can guide the therapeutic approach in terms of diagnostic modality and for following up response to therapy.
- Salivary miR-9, miR-191, and miR-134 in patients with HNSCC serving as biomarkers and provided good discrimination between patients and controls.[63]
- Cell-free DNA has been shown to be effective in diagnosing HNSCC through using liquid biopsy to detect circulation tumor DNA (ctDNA). Tumor cells release DNA when they undergo apoptosis or necrosis.[64] Such modality can be used in various aspects of HNSCC management including diagnosing early-stage disease, monitoring response to therapy, and up to mapping resistance and tumor heterogeneity.[65,66]

SUMMARY

The modern clinical practice of head and neck oncology nearly mandates PET/CT be performed on patients at the time of diagnosis, treatment decision-making, and surveillance of HNSCC. The settings in which head and neck cancer PET/CT are clearly beneficial are in occult primary, advanced disease, and 12 weeks response assessment after definitive chemotherapy and radiation. PET/CT provides additional information that has contributed to improving cancer outcomes by guiding higher intensity treatments to cancer areas while reducing treatments to nonmalignant areas. The future of PET/CT specifically and nuclear medicine broadly in HNSCC is literally and figuratively bright: with more advanced tracer technology, clinical trials of interim PET, and therapeutic application of compounds that directly attach to and destroy cancer cells.

Images on the screen of anatomic and metabolic radiographic aberrations can never adequately capture the social stigma, alienation, and pain that patients suffer after developing head and neck cancers. However, there is no doubt that advances in nuclear medicine are reducing the horrific personal and public health burden of this disease and minimizing the side effects of our intensive treatments. These advances in PET/CT have already provided tangible benefits to patients who now recover faster with fewer irreversible toxicities and are more likely to achieve freedom from recurrent head and neck cancer, for which there are few curative treatment options.

FUNDING

N.D.S. was supported by the National Institutes of Health Director's Early Independence Award DP5 (DP5OD031846) and National Cancer Institute F99/K00 Predoctoral to Postdoctoral Fellow Transition Award (K00CA234954).

CLINICS CARE POINTS

- Diagnostic PET CT is recommended for occult primary tumors, midline tumors, >T2 primary and to assess possibility of distant metastases.
- PET CT is not routinely ordered in patients who have undergone definitive surgery for head and neck squamous cell cancer.
- Early PET CT after head and neck chemoradiation is not indicated due to risk of false positives from inflammation-most are performed 12 weeks post radiation.

REFERENCES

1. Bray F, Ferlay J, Soerjomataram I, et al. Global cancer statistics 2018: GLOBOCAN estimates of incidence and mortality worldwide for 36 cancers in 185 countries. CA: A Cancer J clinicians 2018; 68(6):394–424.
2. Siegel RA-O, Miller KA-O, Fuchs HE, et al. Cancer statistics. CA Cancer J Clin 2021;1542–4863 (Electronic)).
3. Patterson RH, Fischman VG, Wasserman I, et al. Global burden of head and neck cancer: Economic Consequences, health, and the role of surgery. Otolaryngol–Head Neck Surg 2020;162(3):296–303.
4. Park A, Alabaster A, Shen H, et al. Undertreatment of women with locoregionally advanced head and neck cancer. Cancer 2019;125(17):3033–9.
5. Chung CH, Ely K, McGavran L, et al. Increased epidermal growth factor receptor gene copy number is associated with poor prognosis in head and neck squamous cell carcinomas. J Clin Oncol 2006; 24(25):4170–6.
6. Wald T, Birnbaum K, Wiegand S, et al. [Automatic calculation and visualization of comorbidity scores for decision-making in tumor boards]. Laryngo-rhino- otologie 2020;99(1):31–6.
7. Institute NC. SEER-Medicare Data Cost Calculator. 2021. Available at: https://healthcaredelivery.cancer.gov/seermedicare/obtain/costcalc.html.
8. Khan SA, Pruitt SL, Xuan L, et al. How does autoimmune disease impact treatment and outcomes among patients with lung cancer? A national SEER-Medicare analysis. Lung Cancer (Amsterdam, Netherlands) 2018;115:97–102.
9. Khan SA, Pruitt SL, Xuan L, et al. Prevalence of autoimmune disease among patients with lung cancer: Implications for Immunotherapy treatment options. JAMA Oncol 2016;2(11):1507–8.
10. Strojan P, Hutcheson KA, Eisbruch A, et al. Treatment of late sequelae after radiotherapy for head and neck cancer. Cancer Treat Rev 2017;59:79–92.
11. Pfister DG, Spencer S, Adelstein D, et al. Head and neck cancers, version 2.2020, NCCN clinical practice guidelines in oncology. J Natl Compr Canc Netw 2020;18(7):873–98.
12. Abreu C, Grilo A, Lucena F, et al. Oncological patient Anxiety in imaging studies: the PET/CT example. J Cancer Educ 2017;32(4):820–6.
13. Kim S, Oh S, Kim JS, et al. Prognostic value of FDG PET/CT during radiotherapy in head and neck cancer patients. Radiat Oncol J 2018;36(2):95–102.
14. Cooper JS, Pajak TF, Forastiere AA, et al. Postoperative concurrent radiotherapy and chemotherapy for high-risk squamous-cell carcinoma of the head and neck. New Engl J Med 2004;350(19):1937–44.
15. Bernier J, Domenge C, Ozsahin M, et al. Postoperative irradiation with or without Concomitant

chemotherapy for locally advanced head and neck cancer. New Engl J Med 2004;350(19):1945–52.

16. Adeyemi BF, Adekunle LV, Kolude BM, et al. Head and neck cancer–a clinicopathological study in a tertiary care center. J Natl Med Assoc 2008;100(6):690–7.

17. Ologe FE, Adeniji KA, Segun-Busari S. Clinicopathological study of head and neck cancers in Ilorin, Nigeria. Trop doctor 2005;35(1):2–4.

18. Chung CH, Gillison ML. Human papillomavirus in head and neck cancer: its role in Pathogenesis and clinical Implications. Clin Cancer Res 2009; 15(22):6758.

19. Rampias T, Sasaki C, Weinberger P, et al. E6 and E7 gene Silencing and Transformed Phenotype of human papillomavirus 16–positive oropharyngeal cancer cells. JNCI: J Natl Cancer Inst 2009;101(6):412–23.

20. Broski SM, Hunt CH, Johnson GB, et al. The added value of 18F-FDG PET/CT for evaluation of patients with esthesioneuroblastoma. J Nucl Med 2012; 53(8):1200–6.

21. Stroobants S, Verschakelen J, Vansteenkiste J. Value of FDG-PET in the management of non-small cell lung cancer. Eur J Radiol 2003;45(1):49–59.

22. Morris LG, Sikora AG, Patel SG, et al. Second primary cancers after an index head and neck cancer: subsite-specific trends in the era of human papillomavirus-associated oropharyngeal cancer. J Clin Oncol 2011;29(6):739–46.

23. Merino OR, Lindberg RD, Fletcher GH. An analysis of distant metastases from squamous cell carcinoma of the upper respiratory and digestive tracts. Cancer 1977;40(1):145–51.

24. Chen PG, Schoeff SS, Watts CA, et al. Utility of abdominal imaging to assess for liver metastasis in patients with head and neck cancer and abnormal liver function tests. Am J Otolaryngol 2014;35(2): 137–40.

25. Yankevich U, Hughes MA, Rath TJ, et al. PET/CT for head and neck squamous cell carcinoma: should We routinely include the head and abdomen? AJR Am J Roentgenol 2017;208(4):844–8.

26. Castaldi P, Leccisotti L, Bussu F, et al. Role of (18) F-FDG PET-CT in head and neck squamous cell carcinoma. Acta Otorhinolaryngol Ital 2013;33(1): 1–8.

27. National Comprehensive Cancer Network. NCCN Clinical Practice Guidelines in Oncology. 2021.

28. Paleri V, Urbano TG, Mehanna H, et al. Management of neck metastases in head and neck cancer: United Kingdom National Multidisciplinary Guidelines. J Laryngol otology 2016;130(S2):S161–9.

29. Goel R, Moore W, Sumer B, et al. Clinical practice in PET/CT for the management of head and neck squamous cell cancer. AJR Am J roentgenology 2017; 209(2):289–303.

30. Miller FR, Hussey D, Beeram M, et al. Positron emission tomography in the management of Unknown primary head and neck carcinoma. Arch Otolaryngol–Head Neck Surg 2005;131(7):626–9.

31. Pereira G, Silva JC, Monteiro E. Positron emission tomography in the detection of occult primary head and neck carcinoma: a retrospective study. Head neck Oncol 2012;4:34.

32. Mak D, Corry J, Lau E, et al. Role of FDG-PET/CT in staging and follow-up of head and neck squamous cell carcinoma. Q J Nucl Med Mol Imaging 2011; 55(5):487–99.

33. Buchbender C, Heusner TA, Lauenstein TC, et al. Oncologic PET/MRI, part 1: tumors of the brain, head and neck, chest, abdomen, and pelvis. J Nucl Med 2012;53(6):928–38.

34. Laubenbacher C, Saumweber D, Wagner-Manslau C, et al. Comparison of fluorine-18-fluorodeoxyglucose PET, MRI and endoscopy for staging head and neck squamous-cell carcinomas. J Nucl Med 1995;36(10): 1747–57.

35. Boellaard R, Delgado-Bolton R, Oyen WJ, et al. Fdg PET/CT: EANM procedure guidelines for tumour imaging: version 2.0. Eur J Nucl Med Mol Imaging 2015;42(2):328–54.

36. Subramaniam RM, Suarez-Cuervo C, Wilson RF, et al. Effectiveness of prevention Strategies for contrast-induced nephropathy: a systematic review and Meta-analysis. Ann Intern Med 2016;164(6): 406–16.

37. Grégoire V, Chiti A. Molecular imaging in radiotherapy planning for head and neck tumors. J Nucl Med 2011;52(3):331–4.

38. Newbold K, Powell C. PET/CT in radiotherapy planning for head and neck cancer. Front Oncol 2012; 2:189.

39. Goerres GW, Schmid DT, Bandhauer F, et al. Positron emission tomography in the early follow-up of advanced head and neck cancer. Arch Otolaryngol–Head Neck Surg 2004;130(1):105–9.

40. Porceddu SV, Jarmolowski E, Hicks RJ, et al. Utility of positron emission tomography for the detection of disease in residual neck nodes after (chemo) radiotherapy in head and neck cancer. Head & neck 2005;27(3):175–81.

41. Yao M, Smith RB, Graham MM, et al. The role of FDG PET in management of neck metastasis from head-and-neck cancer after definitive radiation treatment. Int J Radiat Oncol Biol Phys 2005;63(4):991–9.

42. Greven KM, Williams DW 3rd, McGuirt WF, et al. Serial positron emission tomography scans following radiation therapy of patients with head and neck cancer. Head & neck 2001;23(11):942–6.

43. Burtness B, Harrington KJ, Greil R, et al. Pembrolizumab alone or with chemotherapy versus cetuximab with chemotherapy for recurrent or metastatic squamous cell carcinoma of the head and neck (KEYNOTE-048): a randomised, open-label, phase 3 study. Lancet (London, England) 2019;394(10212):1915–28.

44. Ferris RL, Blumenschein G, Fayette J, et al. Nivolumab for recurrent squamous-cell carcinoma of the head and neck. New Engl J Med 2016;375(19):1856–67.

45. Mehra R, Huang H, Seal B, et al. Real-world treatment patterns for patients with metastatic head and neck squamous cell carcinoma treated with immuno-oncology therapy. Head & neck 2020; 42(8):2030–8.

46. Merck Sharp & Dohme Corp. GUIDE TO SCORING PD-L1 EXPRESSION USING COMBINED POSITIVE SCORE (CPS). 2021.

47. (FDA) FaDA. FDA approves pembrolizumab for first-line treatment of head and neck squamous cell carcinoma. 2019.

48. Le Gouill S, Casasnovas R-O. Interim PET-driven strategy in de novo diffuse large B-cell lymphoma: do we trust the driver? Blood 2017;129(23): 3059–70.

49. Marcus C, Ciarallo A, Tahari AK, et al. Head and neck PET/CT: therapy response interpretation criteria (Hopkins Criteria)-interreader reliability, accuracy, and survival outcomes. J Nucl Med 2014; 55(9):1411–6.

50. Kendi AT, Brandon D, Switchenko J, et al. Head and neck PET/CT therapy response interpretation criteria (Hopkins criteria) - external validation study. Am J Nucl Med Mol Imaging 2017;7(4):174–80.

51. Marur S, Li S, Cmelak AJ, et al. E1308: phase II trial of Induction chemotherapy followed by reduced-dose radiation and weekly cetuximab in patients with HPV-associated Resectable squamous cell carcinoma of the Oropharynx— ECOG-ACRIN cancer research group. J Clin Oncol 2016;35(5):490–7.

52. Cremonesi M, Garibaldi C, Timmerman R, et al. Interim (18)F-FDG-PET/CT during chemo-radiotherapy in the management of oesophageal cancer patients. A systematic review. Radiother Oncol 2017;125(2):200–12.

53. Marcus C, Subramaniam RM. Role of non-FDG-PET/CT in head and neck cancer. Semin Nucl Med 2021; 51(1):68–78.

54. Bhattacharyya S, Kurdziel K, Wei L, et al. Zirconium-89 labeled panitumumab: a potential immuno-PET probe for HER1-expressing carcinomas. Nucl Med Biol 2013;40(4):451–7.

55. Krishnan G, van den Berg NS, Nishio N, et al. Metastatic and sentinel lymph node mapping using intravenously delivered Panitumumab-IRDye800CW. Theranostics 2021;11(15):7188–98.

56. Colevas AD, Bedi N, Chang S, et al. A study to evaluate immunological response to PD-1 inhibition in squamous cell carcinoma of the head and neck (SCCHN) using novel PET imaging with [18F]F-AraG. J Clin Oncol 2018;36(15_suppl):6050.

57. Keshavarz P, Yazdanpanah F, Rafiee F, et al. Lymphadenopathy following COVID-19 vaccination: imaging findings review. Acad Radiol 2021;28(8): 1058–71.

58. McIntosh LJ, Bankier AA, Vijayaraghavan GR, et al. COVID-19 vaccination-related uptake on FDG PET/CT: an emerging Dilemma and Suggestions for management. AJR Am J roentgenology 2021;186–91.

59. Janssen I, Chen CC, Taieb D, et al. 68Ga-DOTATATE PET/CT in the localization of head and neck paragangliomas compared with other functional imaging modalities and CT/MRI. J Nucl Med 2016;57(2): 186–91.

60. Hofman MS, Lau WF, Hicks RJ. Somatostatin receptor imaging with 68Ga DOTATATE PET/CT: clinical utility, normal patterns, pearls, and pitfalls in interpretation. Radiographics 2015;35(2):500–16.

61. Liu KY, Goldrich DY, Ninan SJ, et al. The value of (68) Gallium-DOTATATE PET/CT in sinonasal neuroendocrine tumor management: a case series. Head & neck 2021;43(6):E30–40.

62. Demokan S, Chang X, Chuang A, et al. KIF1A and EDNRB are differentially methylated in primary HNSCC and salivary rinses. Int J Cancer 2010; 127(10):2351–9.

63. Salazar C, Nagadia R, Pandit P, et al. A novel saliva-based microRNA biomarker panel to detect head and neck cancers. Cell Oncol (Dordrecht) 2014; 37(5):331–8.

64. Stroun M, Lyautey J, Lederrey C, et al. About the possible origin and mechanism of circulating DNA apoptosis and active DNA release. Clin Chim Acta 2001;313(1–2):139–42.

65. Merker JD, Oxnard GR, Compton C, et al. Circulating tumor DNA analysis in patients with cancer: American Society of clinical oncology and College of American Pathologists joint review. J Clin Oncol 2018;36(16):1631–41.

66. Amin MB, Greene FL, Edge SB, et al. The Eighth Edition AJCC Cancer Staging Manual: Continuing to build a bridge from a population-based to a more "personalized" approach to cancer staging. CA: a Cancer J clinicians 2017;67(2):93–9.

PET Imaging of Oral Cavity and Oropharyngeal Cancers

Charles Marcus, MD[a],*, Rathan M. Subramaniam, MD, PhD, MPH, MBA[b]

KEYWORDS

- FDG PET • PET/CT • Oral cavity cancer • Oropharyngeal cancer • Neoplasm • Staging

KEY POINTS

- Fluorine-18 fluorodeoxyglucose PET/computed tomography (^{18}F-FDG PET/CT) plays an important role in staging, treatment planning, treatment response assessment, recurrent disease detection, and prognosis prediction in oral cavity and oropharyngeal cancers.
- ^{18}F-FDG PET/CT is superior to conventional imaging modalities in the detection of disease, especially nodal and distant metastatic disease.
- ^{18}F-FDG PET/MR evidence in the evaluation of these cancers is constantly evolving. PET/MR provides superior soft tissue contrast and can add value in the evaluation of these primary tumors.

INTRODUCTION

Head and neck cancer is a common malignancy encountered in every molecular imaging practice. These cancers commonly arise from the squamous cells lining the mucosa and are termed squamous cell carcinoma (SCC). These cancers are more common in patients 50 years or older, and White men. The most common site of head and neck SCC (HNSCC) is the oropharynx (31%), followed by the oral cavity (29%) and larynx (29%).[1] In 2020, 53,260 new cases of oral cavity and oropharyngeal cancers were estimated in the United States, accounting for 2.9% of all new cases. The estimated number of deaths attributed to this malignancy was 10,750, accounting for 1.8% of all cancer deaths. The outcome of these patients varies by stage and accurate diagnosis, staging and appropriate treatment is crucial to improve patient prognosis. The overall 5-year survival in these patients is 66%, ranging from 85% in localized disease to 40% in patients with distant disease.[2] Cancers of the oral cavity include cancers involving the buccal mucosa, floor of mouth, anterior tongue, alveolar ridge, retromolar trigone, and hard palate. Cancers of the oropharynx include cancers of the tongue base, tonsils, posterior pharyngeal wall, and soft palate (National Comprehensive Cancer Network [NCCN] v1.2021).[3]

Fluorine-18 fluorodeoxyglucose PET/computed tomography (^{18}F-FDG PET/CT) has become an important modality in the diagnosis, staging, restaging, follow-up, treatment planning, treatment response assessment, and prognosis prediction in patients with oral cavity and oropharyngeal SCC (OPSCC). This article reviews the current role of ^{18}F-FDG PET/CT in the evaluation and management of oral cavity and OPSCC. Recent advances in ^{18}F-FDG PET/MR imaging clinical use is also reviewed briefly.

[a] Division of Nuclear Medicine and Molecular Imaging, Department of Radiology and Imaging Services, Emory University Hospital, 1364 Clifton Road NE, 1st FL #E163, Atlanta, GA 30322, USA; [b] Dean's Office, Otago Medical School, University of Otago, Dunedin, New Zealand
* Corresponding author. Division of Nuclear Medicine and Molecular Imaging, Department of Radiology and Imaging Services, 1364 Clifton Road NE, 1st FL #E163, Atlanta, GA 30322.
E-mail address: charlesmarcus1986@gmail.com

PET Clin 17 (2022) 223–234
https://doi.org/10.1016/j.cpet.2021.12.005
1556-8598/22/© 2021 Elsevier Inc. All rights reserved.

STAGING ORAL CAVITY AND OROPHARYNGEAL SQUAMOUS CELL CARCINOMA

Staging of these tumors has evolved significantly over the years. Human papilloma virus (HPV) or p16 association has become an important component of the evaluation and characterization of these cancers, including staging. The widely used staging system incorporates the primary tumor characteristics (T), nodal disease (N), and metastases (M), as outlined by the American Joint Committee on Cancer system, most recently updated in January 2018.[4] Detailed review of the staging system is beyond the scope of this article. Salient features to evaluate on imaging are highlighted in the following sections. While evaluating the tumor, features to be noted are tumor size in the longest dimension, and extension of tumor into adjacent structures. Perineural spread of tumor should be actively incorporated into the primary tumor evaluation, because it can affect treatment planning, best evaluated on MR imaging but can be seen on ^{18}F-FDG PET/CT.[5] Limitations of imaging in distinguishing certain primary tumor characteristics should be understood, such as depth of invasion, which is best evaluated histopathologically. Careful evaluation of nodal metastasis is very important for treatment planning and outcome. If nodal disease is identified, whether the affected node is ipsilateral or contralateral to the side of the primary tumor, size of the abnormal node, level of the node, and any extranodal extension of tumor. The evaluation of extranodal extension is limited on PET/CT.[6] HPV-negative tumors have poor prognosis in comparison with HPV-associated primary tumors, and this is taken into consideration and the staging varies accordingly. For example, a 4-cm p16 positive primary oropharyngeal tumor with no nodal disease is staged as stage I, whereas a 4-cm p16 negative primary oropharyngeal tumor with no nodal disease is staged as stage II. Clear advantage of ^{18}F-FDG PET/CT over other conventional imaging methods is the identification of distant metastatic disease and should be carefully evaluated in staging these patients.[7]

IMAGING FINDINGS

In the initial workup, ^{18}F-FDG PET/CT is considered in the evaluation of nodal disease in patients with multiple nodal level or lower level nodal involvement, and/or high-grade tumors. In patients with occult primary malignancy not identified on conventional imaging, ^{18}F-FDG PET/CT can be used to localize the site of primary disease before any intervention, biopsy, or examination under anesthesia. ^{18}F-FDG PET/CT is also considered for the evaluation of distant metastatic disease in patients with larger tumors (T3-T4) and/or with nodal metastases ($\geq$N1 disease) (NCCN Guidelines Version 1.2021).[3]

PRIMARY TUMOR STAGING

Although the role of ^{18}F-FDG PET/CT in the evaluation of the primary tumor is somewhat limited, when combined with a contrast-enhanced CT of the head and neck, it can have high sensitivity (96%).[8] ^{18}F-FDG PET/CT is especially useful in primary tumor evaluation in patients with dental or metallic implants that cause significant artifact, resulting in suboptimal evaluation on MR imaging ($P = .004$). In these patients, the findings on PET/CT correlated better with pathologic tumor volume than MR imaging.[9] In the evaluation of bone marrow invasion of adjacent osseous structures such as the maxilla and mandible, MR imaging is more sensitive (97% vs 78%) with high negative predictive value (98% vs 89%). However, ^{18}F-FDG PET/CT can play a complementary role in patients with findings of bone marrow invasion on MR imaging with higher specificity (83% vs 61%) and positive predictive value (69% vs 55%), to exclude false positive findings.[10] In all different T stages, ^{18}F-FDG PET/CT has been shown to have higher diagnostic performance than conventional imaging methods such as CT or MR imaging (98% vs 88%) in HNSCC, most of which included oral cavity and oropharyngeal tumors.[11] In smaller tumors (T1-T2), ^{18}F-FDG PET/CT has been shown to identify more lesions in the oral cavity and oropharynx, not discernible on MR imaging, attributed to the high metabolic activity seen in these SCCs with high soft tissue contrast, despite lower spatial resolution.[12]

STAGING CERVICAL NODAL METASTASES

In staging oral cavity and oropharyngeal cancer, ^{18}F-FDG PET/CT is valuable in detecting clinically negative nodal metastases, which has a significant impact on treatment planning. Recently published data from a multicenter prospective clinical trial (ACRIN 6685), composed mostly of oral cavity and pharyngeal SCC, show that preoperative staging with ^{18}F-FDG PET/CT of clinically N0 patients with T2-T4 disease, had a high negative predictive value of 86% by qualitative visual assessment and 94% with a maximum standardized uptake value (SUVmax) cutoff of 1.8. These findings lead to change in surgical management in 22% of the patients, resulting in additional neck dissections in 14% of the patients and fewer neck dissections in 5%.[13] Even in smaller tumors (T1-T2), the specificity appears to be high (98%), even though the sensitivity was low (21%), detecting occult metastases in 14% of the patients.[14] The PET/CT findings appear to vary depending on the HPV status of the patients, with HPV-associated nodal metastases demonstrating significantly higher FDG avidity (P < .01).[15] In patients with clinically node-negative assessments, the ACRIN 6685 study analysis demonstrated higher risk of PET/CT-detected nodal metastases in the ipsilateral level I for oral cavity tumors and level IIa for oropharyngeal tumors. This should be considered in the imaging search pattern and treatment planning of these patients[16] (**Fig. 1**).

STAGING DISTANT DISEASE AND DETECTION OF A SECOND PRIMARY MALIGNANCY

In patients with HNSCC, composed of oral cavity and oropharyngeal tumors mostly, distant disease or a second primary malignancy was detected more commonly in advanced tumors (T3-T4) and in patients with history of smoking who underwent ^{18}F-FDG PET/CT/MR imaging. Second primary cancer was detected in as many as 12% of the patients.[17] Distant metastatic disease has been diagnosed in approximately 10% of the patients, predominantly in the lungs, followed by liver and bones. The reported sensitivity, specificity, and positive predictive values were 97%, 95%, and 67%, respectively. The incidence of distant metastases is less common in oral cavity and oropharyngeal tumors in comparison with hypopharyngeal or laryngeal cancers and patients with metastatic disease in lower neck nodes (IV, VB). Distant metastatic disease as expected can have a negative impact on patient outcome with lower 5-year overall survival (12% vs 82%; P < .001). These findings show the importance of accurate detection of distant metastatic disease in these patients to guide optimal management to improve patient prognosis.[18] ^{18}F-FDG PET/CT has the most value in distant disease detection in comparison with conventional imaging techniques, given the ability to image the whole body in one sitting.

ROLE IN TREATMENT PLANNING

Incorporation of ^{18}F-FDG PET/CT findings in treatment planning has become more prevalent in the recent past, especially in radiation treatment planning, which typically used CT and/or MR imaging findings. ^{18}F-FDG PET/CT findings can change the TNM staging in as many as 48% of the patients, modifying radiation therapy planning in up to 68% of patients with HNSCC.[19] The goal of an optimal radiation treatment plan is to provide adequate dose to the tumor while keeping dose to the surrounding normal tissues as minimal as possible to reduce adverse effects. A prospective multicenter study showed smaller tumor volumes in HNSCC, especially in oropharyngeal tumors (P < .0001), in comparison with CT-guided volume estimation, PET/CT-guided estimation resulted in reduced nontarget radiation dose to salivary glands and the oral cavity. This method also showed good nodal disease control on subsequent neck dissections.[20] In comparison with CT-guided techniques, the use of ^{18}F-FDG PET/CT has shown to change treatment volumes in one-fourth of patients with oral cavity cancers.[21] Using ^{18}F-FDG PET/CT-based intensity modulation arc radiation therapy in comparison with the conventional intensity modulation radiation therapy has shown to improve dose delivery to the tumor while decreasing radiation to normal surrounding tissues.[22] The different PET/CT techniques and parameters used for treatment planning are constantly evolving. For example, a multicenter study of patients with head and neck cancer found that using the ratio of tumor to cervical spinal cord uptake instead of the more commonly SUVmax resulted in better reproducibility for radiation treatment planning.[23] However, more studies are warranted to validate these findings.

TREATMENT RESPONSE ASSESSMENT AND PROGNOSIS

It is well known that ^{18}F-FDG PET/CT plays an important role in treatment assessment in patients with oral cavity and OPSCC. As mentioned earlier, the optimal time interval to perform these studies for treatment response assessment is 3 to 6 months after treatment completion, especially after radiation therapy to decrease false positive and inconclusive results related to inflammatory radiotracer uptake in the treatment bed.[24] A meta-analysis of 22 studies has shown an overall sensitivity, specificity, and positive and negative predictive values of 85%, 93%, 58%, and 100%, respectively, with lower sensitivity and specificity associated with HPV-associated tumors.[25] As seen, studies report lower positive predictive value, especially in studies done before 12 weeks of treatment completion (P = .06) and in HPV-associated tumors (P = .01). As expected, patients with good response to treatment have better

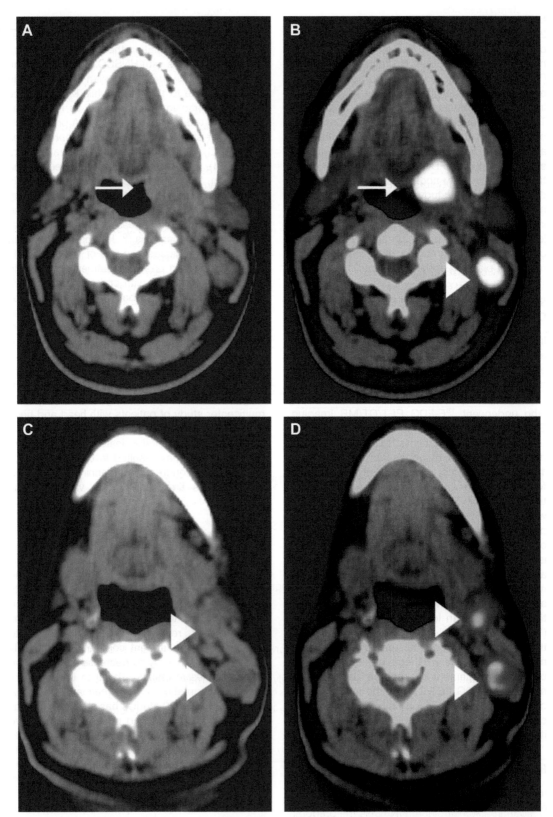

Fig. 1. A 60-year-old man with recently diagnosed HPV-positive SCC of the left tonsil. Axial CT (*A, C*), axial fused PET/CT (*B, D*) of the staging ^{18}F-FDG PET/CT demonstrates FDG-avid left tonsillar mass (SUVmax 14.6) (*white arrows*) and metastatic partially cystic left level 2 cervical lymphadenopathy (SUVmax 16.5) (*white arrowheads*). Patient underwent left transoral robotic surgery with left neck dissection and adjuvant radiation.

Table 1
Hopkins qualitative treatment response criteria

Score	Fluorine-18-Fluorodeoxyglucose Uptake	Response Category
1	Uptake less than internal jugular vein (IJV)	Complete metabolic response
2	Focal uptake greater than IJV but less than liver	Likely complete metabolic response
3	Diffuse uptake greater than IJV or liver	Likely inflammation
4	Focal uptake greater than liver	Likely residual disease
5	Focal and intense uptake greater than liver	Residual disease

outcome (87% vs 51% 5-year overall survival; $P \leq .001$).[26] A first posttreatment PET/CT that shows no significant metabolically active residual disease is associated with longer overall and progression-free survival.[27]

^{18}F-FDG PET/CT can also diagnose nodal disease in patients treated with primary radiation therapy, thereby identifying patients who could benefit from neck dissections, decreasing the rates of unnecessary neck dissections. This can decrease the side effects, costs, and comorbidities associated with these surgical procedures.[28,29] In patients with incomplete disease response without compelling imaging findings of residual disease, a second-look PET/CT may be of benefit and can decrease the rates of salvage neck dissections.[30] A study of predominantly patients with OPSCC, evaluating the use of a

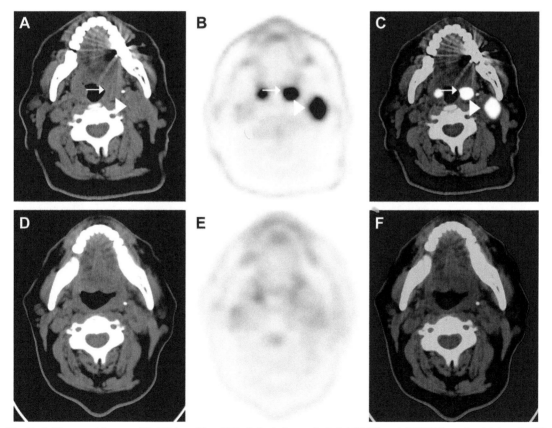

Fig. 2. A 52-year-old man with HPV-positive SCC of the left tonsil. Axial CT (*A*), axial PET (*B*), and axial fused PET/CT (*C*) of a staging ^{18}F-FDG PET/CT demonstrates an intensely FDG-avid left tonsil lesion (*white arrows*) with an SUVmax of 24.1 with metastatic left level 2A cervical lymphadenopathy (*white arrowhead*) (Hopkins Score 5). Approximately 12 weeks after completion of primary chemoradiation therapy, the axial CT (*D*), axial PET (*E*), and axial fused PET/CT (*F*) of the restaging PET/CT demonstrates complete metabolic response (Hopkins Score 1).

second-look PET/CT after an initial treatment response assessment scan showing incomplete response performed approximately 3 months after the prior scan, showed complete response in more than half the patients (60%). None of these patients demonstrated disease progression at follow-up.[31]

In recent years, qualitative response criteria have gained interest in the evaluation of treatment response in HNSCC. These response criteria use qualitative comparison of metabolic activity within the tumor or lymph nodes to reference background blood pool and the liver to assign scores and evaluate their ability to predict the possibility of residual disease. For example, the Hopkins criteria uses a 5-point scale (**Table 1**) and has been evaluated in HNSCC, predominantly in patients with OPSCC (63%) who were treated with radiation or chemoradiation. The criteria demonstrated high negative predictive value (92%) and accuracy (87%). There was also significant association with progression-free and overall survival. The internal jugular vein (IJV)

was used as the blood pool reference, because certain head and neck (PET/CT) protocols have a separate head and neck acquisition.[32] An external validation study showed that the criteria had a sensitivity, specificity, and positive and negative predictive value of 67%, 87%, 33%, and 97%, respectively, with ability to predict progression-free survival and had high interreader agreement.[33] In patients with residual neck nodes after completion of definitive chemoradiation, the Hopkins criteria was able to predict outcome, which may be useful in identifying patients who would benefit from adjuvant treatment[34] (**Fig. 2**). Other response criteria have also been studied in assessing treatment response, such as the Porceddu, Deauville, and Neck Imaging Reporting and Data System (NI-RADS) criteria. A comparative study showed that all these criteria appear to demonstrate good diagnostic performance in detecting residual disease and predicting progression-free survival ($P < .001$). Although the number of indeterminate results was higher with NI-RADS and Porceddu criteria, the

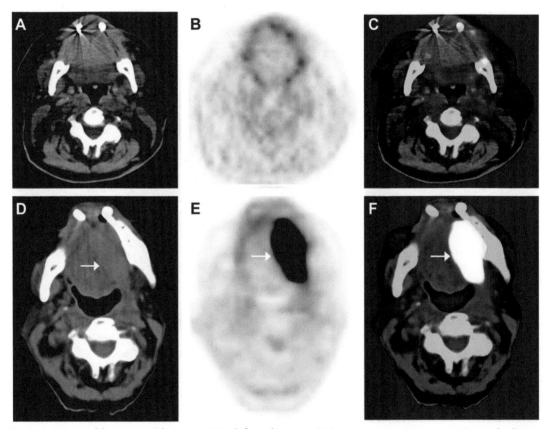

Fig. 3. A 74-year-old woman with HPV-positive left oral tongue SCC, status post primary resection and adjuvant radiation. Axial CT (*A*), axial PET (*B*), and axial fused PET/CT (*C*) of a posttreatment ^{18}F-FDG PET/CT demonstrates no hypermetabolic focus, compatible with complete metabolic response. Axial CT (*D*), axial PET (*E*), and axial fused PET/CT (*F*) of a restaging PET/CT demonstrates a large recurrent left oral tongue mass (*white arrows*) with intense metabolic activity (SUVmax 26.7).

investigators found that the Porceddu and Deauville criteria appeared to maintain a high negative predictive value while keeping the number of indeterminate results low.[35] The more widely used Response Evaluation Criteria in Solid Tumors (RECIST) and PET Response Criteria in Solid Tumors (PERCIST) for treatment response assessment in oncologic imaging have also been applied to HNSCC. Although the study reported lower diagnostic performance (negative predictive value 78%) than the qualitative criteria discussed previously, combing RECIST and PERCIST improved the detection of residual nodal disease.[36] Patients with complete response using PERCIST criteria showed better progression-free and overall survival, $P < .0001$).[37]

Evaluation of Recurrent Disease

In patients with advanced head and neck cancer who are treated with primary surgery with or without adjuvant treatment, results of ^{18}F-FDG PET/CT performed 6 months after primary treatment was predictive of recurrent disease and

overall survival (23% vs 82% and 48% vs 92%, respectively). Histopathological features such as nodal disease, extranodal extension, positive margins, and perineural invasion were associated with metabolically active recurrent disease ($P < .05$).[38] PET/CT findings in the evaluation of these patients with recurrent HNSCC, can modify the treatment plan in comparison with conventional imaging techniques in as many as one-third of patients ($P < .001$).[39] Although routine follow-up or surveillance ^{18}F-FDG PET/CT may not be applicable in all patients, in patients with increased risk of recurrent disease, such as larger tumors, nodal metastases, tumor depth ≥ 10 mm, or perineural, lymphatic, or vascular invasion, it can be a valuable tool for identifying recurrence with impact on patient outcome.[40] Following primary surgical resection and reconstruction, ^{18}F-FDG PET combined with contrast-enhanced CT has shown to have good diagnostic performance in detecting local disease recurrence.[41] A meta-analysis of 27 prospective studies with pathology or clinical

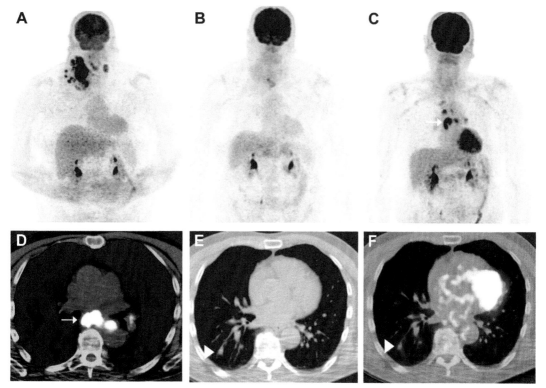

Fig. 4. A 60-year-old man with HPV-associated metastatic SCC of the right tongue base. Coronal maximum intensity projection (MIP) (*A*) of a staging ^{18}F-FDG PET/CT demonstrates a right tongue base lesion with extensive bilateral cervical nodal metastases. Coronal MIP (*B*) of a posttreatment PET/CT following chemoradiation demonstrates interval favorable response to treatment. Coronal MIP (*C*), axial fused PET/CT (*D*), axial CT (*E*), and axial fused PET/CT (*F*) of a follow-up PET/CT approximately 1 year after treatment completion demonstrates hypermetabolic mediastinal lymphadenopathy (*white arrows*) and a mildly hypermetabolic right lower lobe lung nodule (*white arrowheads*). Bronchoscopy and biopsy of the lung nodule demonstrated metastatic SCC.

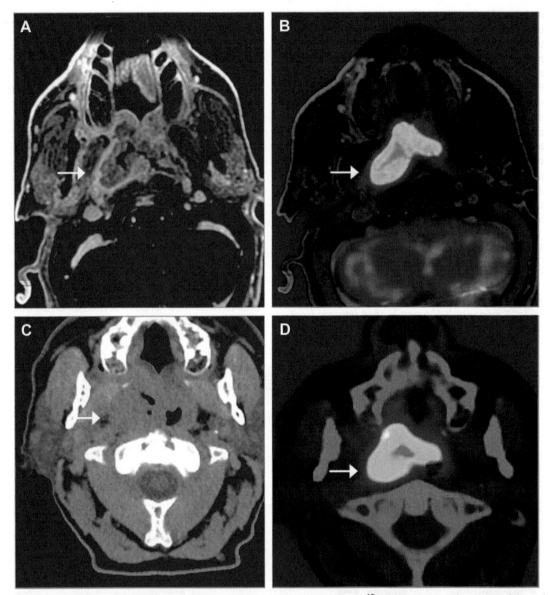

Fig. 5. Axial postcontrast T1-weighted fat-suppressed MR (*A*), axial fused ^{18}F-FDG PET/MR (*B*), axial CT (*C*), and axial fused ^{18}F-FDG PET/CT (*D*) images showing an hypermetabolic OPSCC tumor (*white arrows*) extending superiorly to involve the nasopharynx. The soft tissue delineation and soft tissue contrast is superior on the PET/MR images in comparison with PET/CT.

follow-up correlation demonstrated pooled sensitivity and specificity of 86%, 82% for the primary tumor site, 72%, 88% for nodal metastasis, and 85%, 95%, respectively, for distant disease[42] (**Figs. 3** and **4**).

DETECTION OF OCCULT PRIMARY

Localization of clinically unknown head and neck primary malignancy is important for the appropriate treatment planning and to provide best possible outcome. Most of these occult tumors are localized to the pharyngeal tonsils and tongue base in almost half of these patients, and these tumors are detected on ^{18}F-FDG PET/CT in up to 70% of these patients.[43] The reported sensitivity, specificity, and positive and negative predictive value were 100%, 67%, 65%, and 100%, respectively.[44] Normal physiologic radiotracer uptake in the tonsils is often a source of false positive or false negative interpretation of these studies. Careful comparison of asymmetric radiotracer uptake is essential in improving the diagnostic accuracy. Calculating the SUVmax ratio of bilateral tonsillar radiotracer uptake can be helpful. A cutoff ratio of approximately 1.5 has been shown to have excellent sensitivity and specificity (100%). The mean SUVmax of tonsillar malignancy was 9.4 ± 4.5 in comparison with physiologic tonsillar uptake, which was 3.0 ± 1.1, demonstrating the high FDG avidity of these tumors.[45]

PET/MR IMAGING IN ORAL CAVITY AND OROPHARYNGEAL CANCERS

With the recent development of PET/MR imaging technology, it is good to understand the applications of PET/MR in the evaluation of oral cavity and oropharyngeal tumors. Combining the metabolic activity information with the superior soft tissue resolution of MR imaging and the decreased radiation exposure can offer several advantages, especially in local disease characterization.[46,47] The malignant lesion detection/localization of PET/MR is equal to that of PET/CT, with comparable image quality.[48] The acquisition protocol may vary across practices and depends on the experience and comfort of the interpreting physicians. One important component is whether to use gadolinium contrast-enhanced MR imaging with the PET/MR acquisition. A recent study showed no significant difference in the diagnostic accuracy between enhanced and unenhanced imaging techniques ($P < .001$).[49] The MR protocol must be refined for the best possible diagnostic performance. The use of multiparametric MR improves tumor detection rates.[50]

In the evaluation of the primary tumor, PET/MR is especially useful in detecting adjacent structure involvement, given the higher soft tissue resolution (**Fig. 5**). The sensitivity for detecting mandibular and medial pterygoid muscle invasion was high (100%, 83%, respectively). The corresponding specificity is high for muscular invasion (100%) but decreases for osseous invasion (40%). This may be especially useful when the evaluation of osseous invasion can be limited by dental artifact commonly encountered on CT images.[51] These findings can have a significant impact on surgical treatment planning. In detection of nodal metastases, PET/MR may not add value to PET/CT.[52,53] Similarly, the detection of distant metastatic disease appears comparable to PET/CT.[54] Information obtained from PET/MR can be used for radiation treatment planning.[55] The metabolic information obtained can be combined with diffusion characteristics for improved radiation treatment planning.[56] In the evaluation of recurrent disease, combining the diffusion restriction and metabolic activity helps in accurate delineation of

the recurrent disease, correlating with pathologic T staging and can be useful in planning salvage treatment in patients treated with primary chemoradiation or radiation therapy.[57]

The literature on ^{18}F-FDG PET/MR is constantly evolving as more centers start establishing these systems and incorporating them into routine clinical use. Currently, it is unclear whether ^{18}F-FDG PET/MR can replace ^{18}F-FDG PET/CT in the evaluation of patients with oral cavity or OPSCC. Larger studies evaluating the role of ^{18}F-FDG PET/MR and comparing it with ^{18}F-FDG PET/CT is warranted.

SUMMARY

^{18}F-FDG PET/CT plays an important role in the staging, treatment planning, treatment response assessment, detection of recurrent disease, and prediction of prognosis in patients with oral cavity and OPSCC. PET/CT has advantage especially in the detection of nodal, distant metastatic disease and second primary malignancy. PET/MR provides superior soft tissue contrast while decreasing radiation exposure, which is advantageous in evaluation of the primary tumor.

CLINICS CARE POINTS

- 18F-FDG PET/CT has the most value in detecting nodal or distant metastases or a second primary malignancy at staging.
- Radiation treatment planning incorporating metabolic findings from 18F-FDG PET/CT has advantages over conventional planning methods.
- 18F-FDG PET/CT guided treatment response assessment has shown to significantly improve patient outcomes.
- In patients with recurrent disease, 18F-FDG PET/CT can have a significant impact on treatment planning and outcomes.
- PET/MR may be useful in select patients with superior soft tissue resolution and offers the benefit of combining the advantage of MR with metabolic information in a single modality.

ACKNOWLEDGMENTS

PET/MR case example, courtesy of Dr Greg Avey, MD, Associate Professor, Department of

Radiology, University of Wisconsin-Madison, Madison, WI.

DISCLOSURE

The authors have nothing to disclose.

REFERENCES

1. Fakhry C, Krapcho M, Eisele DW, et al. Head and neck squamous cell cancers in the United States are rare and the risk now is higher among white individuals compared with black individuals. Cancer 2018;124(10):2125–33.

2. National Cancer Institute. National Cancer Institute: Surveillance, Epidemiology, and End Results Program. Cancer Stat Facts. 2020. Available at: https://seer.cancer.gov/statfacts/. Accessed March 30, 2021.

3. National Comprehensive Cancer Network. NCCN clinical practice guidelines in oncology: head and neck cancers. NCCN Guidel Version 12020. 2020.

4. AJCC. AJCC Cancer staging manual. In: Amin MB, Edge S, Greene F, et al, editors. 8th edition. New York: Springer International Publishing; 2018.

5. Lee H, Lazor JW, Assadsangabi R, et al. An imager's guide to perineural tumor spread in head and neck cancers: radiologic footprints on 18 F-FDG PET, with CT and MRI Correlates. J Nucl Med 2019; 60(3):304–11.

6. Snyder V, Goyal LK, Bowers EMR, et al. PET/CT poorly predicts AJCC 8th Edition pathologic staging in HPV-related oropharyngeal cancer. Laryngoscope 2021. https://doi.org/10.1002/lary.29366.

7. Glastonbury CM. Head and neck squamous cell cancer: approach to staging and surveillance. In: ; 2020:215-222. doi:10.1007/978-3-030-38490-6_17

8. Krabbe CA, Balink H, Roodenburg JLN, et al. Performance of 18F-FDG PET/contrast-enhanced CT in the staging of squamous cell carcinoma of the oral cavity and oropharynx. Int J Oral Maxillofac Surg 2011;40(11):1263–70.

9. Hong HR, Jin S, Koo HJ, et al. Clinical values of 18 F-FDG PET/CT in oral cavity cancer with dental artifacts on CT or MRI. J Surg Oncol 2014;110(6):696–701.

10. Abd El-Hafez YG, Chen C-C, Ng S-H, et al. Comparison of PET/CT and MRI for the detection of bone marrow invasion in patients with squamous cell carcinoma of the oral cavity. Oral Oncol 2011;47(4):288–95.

11. Roh J-L, Yeo N-K, Kim JS, et al. Utility of 2-[18F] fluoro-2-deoxy-d-glucose positron emission tomography and positron emission tomography/computed tomography imaging in the preoperative staging of head and neck squamous cell carcinoma. Oral Oncol 2007;43(9):887–93.

12. Chaput A, Robin P, Podeur F, et al. Diagnostic performance of 18 fluorodesoxyglucose positron emission/computed tomography and magnetic resonance imaging in detecting T1-T2 head and neck squamous cell carcinoma. Laryngoscope 2018;128(2):378–85.

13. Lowe VJ, Duan F, Subramaniam RM, et al. Multicenter trial of [18 F]fluorodeoxyglucose positron emission tomography/computed tomography staging of head and neck cancer and negative predictive value and surgical impact in the N0 Neck: results from ACRIN 6685. J Clin Oncol 2019; 37(20):1704–12.

14. Zhang H, Seikaly H, Biron VL, et al. Utility of PET-CT in detecting nodal metastasis in cN0 early stage oral cavity squamous cell carcinoma. Oral Oncol 2018; 80:89–92.

15. Kendi ATK, Magliocca K, Corey A, et al. Do 18F-FDG PET/CT parameters in oropharyngeal and oral cavity squamous cell carcinomas indicate HPV status? Clin Nucl Med 2015;40(3):e196–200.

16. Stack BC, Duan F, Subramaniam RM, et al. FDG-PET/CT and pathology in newly diagnosed head and neck cancer: ACRIN 6685 Trial, FDG-PET/CT cN0. Otolaryngol Neck Surg 2020. https://doi.org/10.1177/0194599820969104. 019459982096910.

17. Stadler TM, Morand GB, Rupp NJ, et al. FDG-PET-CT/MRI in head and neck squamous cell carcinoma: impact on pretherapeutic N classification, detection of distant metastases, and second primary tumors. Head Neck 2021. https://doi.org/10.1002/hed.26668.

18. Xu G-Z, Guan D-J, He Z-Y. 18FDG-PET/CT for detecting distant metastases and second primary cancers in patients with head and neck cancer. A meta-analysis. Oral Oncol 2011;47(7):560–5.

19. Kandeel A, Saied M, Aldaly M, et al. Impact of 18F-2-fluoro-2-deoxy-D-glucose PET/computerized tomography on the initial staging and changing the management intent in head and neck squamous cell carcinoma. Nucl Med Commun 2021;42(2):216–24.

20. Leclerc M, Lartigau E, Lacornerie T, et al. Primary tumor delineation based on 18FDG PET for locally advanced head and neck cancer treated by chemo-radiotherapy. Radiother Oncol 2015;116(1):87–93.

21. Mazzola R, Alongi P, Ricchetti F, et al. 18F-Fluorodeoxyglucose-PET/CT in locally advanced head and neck cancer can influence the stage migration and nodal radiation treatment volumes. Radiol Med 2017;122(12):952–9.

22. Berwouts D, Olteanu LAM, Speleers B, et al. Intensity modulated arc therapy implementation in a three phase adaptive 18F-FDG-PET voxel intensity-based planning strategy for head-and-neck cancer. Radiat Oncol 2016;11(1):52.

23. van den Bosch S, Dijkema T, Philippens MEP, et al. Tumor to cervical spinal cord standardized uptake ratio (SUR) improves the reproducibility of 18F-FDG-PET based tumor segmentation in head and neck squamous cell carcinoma in a multicenter setting. Radiother Oncol 2019;130:39–45.

24. Heineman TE, Kuan EC, St. John MA. When should surveillance imaging be performed after treatment for head and neck cancer? Laryngoscope 2017; 127(3):533–4.

25. Helsen N, Van den Wyngaert T, Carp L, et al. FDG-PET/CT for treatment response assessment in head and neck squamous cell carcinoma: a systematic review and meta-analysis of diagnostic performance. Eur J Nucl Med Mol Imaging 2018;45(6): 1063–71.

26. Urban R, Godoy T, Olson R, et al. FDG-PET/CT scan assessment of response 12 weeks post radical radiotherapy in oropharynx head and neck cancer: the impact of p16 status. Radiother Oncol 2020; 148:14–20.

27. Ghosh-Laskar S, Mummudi N, Rangarajan V, et al. Prognostic value of response assessment fluorodeoxyglucose positron emission tomography-computed tomography scan in radically treated squamous cell carcinoma of head and neck: long-term results of a prospective study. J Cancer Res Ther 2019;15(3):596.

28. Benjamin J, Hephzibah J, Shanthly N, et al. F-18 FDG PET-CT for response evaluation in head and neck malignancy: experience from a tertiary level hospital in south India. Cancer Rep 2021. https://doi.org/10.1002/cnr2.1333.

29. Mehanna H, McConkey CC, Rahman JK, et al. PET-NECK: a multicentre randomised Phase III non-inferiority trial comparing a positron emission tomography–computerised tomography-guided watch-and-wait policy with planned neck dissection in the management of locally advanced (N2/N3) nodal metastases in. Health Technol Assess (Rockv) 2017;21(17):1–122.

30. Liu HY, Milne R, Lock G, et al. Utility of a repeat PET/CT scan in HPV-associated oropharyngeal cancer following incomplete nodal response from (chemo) radiotherapy. Oral Oncol 2019;88:153–9.

31. Prestwich RJD, Arunsingh M, Zhong J, et al. Second-look PET-CT following an initial incomplete PET-CT response to (chemo)radiotherapy for head and neck squamous cell carcinoma. Eur Radiol 2020;30(2):1212–20.

32. Marcus C, Ciarallo A, Tahari AK, et al. Head and neck PET/CT: therapy response interpretation criteria (Hopkins criteria)–interreader reliability, accuracy, and survival outcomes. J Nucl Med 2014; 55(9):1411–6.

33. Kendi AT, Brandon D, Switchenko J, et al. Head and neck PET/CT therapy response interpretation criteria (Hopkins criteria) - external validation study. Am J Nucl Med Mol Imaging 2017;7(4):174–80. Available at: http://www.ncbi.nlm.nih.gov/pubmed/28913156.

34. Wray R, Sheikhbahaei S, Marcus C, et al. Therapy response assessment and patient outcomes in head and neck squamous cell carcinoma: FDG PET Hopkins criteria versus residual neck node size and morphologic features. Am J Roentgenol 2016;207(3):641–7.

35. Zhong J, Sundersingh M, Dyker K, et al. Post-treatment FDG PET-CT in head and neck carcinoma: comparative analysis of 4 qualitative interpretative criteria in a large patient cohort. Sci Rep 2020;10(1):4086.

36. Kishikawa T, Suzuki M, Takemoto N, et al. Response evaluation criteria in solid tumors (RECIST) and PET response criteria in solid tumors (PERCIST) for response evaluation of the neck after chemoradiotherapy in head and neck squamous cell carcinoma. Head Neck 2021;43(4):1184–93.

37. Katsuura T, Kitajima K, Fujiwara M, et al. Assessment of tumor response to chemoradiotherapy and predicting prognosis in patients with head and neck squamous cell carcinoma by PERCIST. Ann Nucl Med 2018;32(7):453–62.

38. Jung AR, Roh J-L, Kim JS, et al. Post-treatment 18F-FDG PET/CT for predicting survival and recurrence in patients with advanced-stage head and neck cancer undergoing curative surgery. Oral Oncol 2020;107:104750.

39. Rohde M, Nielsen AL, Johansen J, et al. Upfront PET/CT affects management decisions in patients with recurrent head and neck squamous cell carcinoma. Oral Oncol 2019;94:1–7.

40. Lin H-C, Kang C-J, Huang S-F, et al. Clinical impact of PET/CT imaging after adjuvant therapy in patients with oral cavity squamous cell carcinoma. Eur J Nucl Med Mol Imaging 2017;44(10):1702–11.

41. Müller J, Hüllner M, Strobel K, et al. The value of 18 F-FDG-PET/CT imaging in oral cavity cancer patients following surgical reconstruction. Laryngoscope 2015;125(8):1861–8.

42. Cheung PKF, Chin RY, Eslick GD. Detecting residual/recurrent head neck squamous cell carcinomas using PET or PET/CT. Otolaryngol Neck Surg 2016; 154(3):421–32.

43. Kuta V, Williams B, Rigby M, et al. Management of head and neck primary unknown squamous cell carcinoma using combined positron emission tomography-computed tomography and transoral laser microsurgery. Laryngoscope 2018;128(10):2307–11.

44. Ng Shu-Hang, Yen Tzu-Chen, Liao Chun-Ta, et al. 18F-FDG PET and CT/MRI in oral cavity squamous cell carcinoma: a prospective study of 124 patients with histologic correlation. J Nucl Med 2005;46(7): 1136–43.

45. Davison JM, Ozonoff A, Imsande HM, et al. Squamous cell carcinoma of the palatine tonsils: FDG

standardized uptake value ratio as a biomarker to differentiate tonsillar carcinoma from physiologic uptake. Radiology 2010;255(2):578–85.

46. Al-Nabhani KZ, Syed R, Michopoulou S, et al. Qualitative and quantitative comparison of PET/CT and PET/MR imaging in clinical practice. J Nucl Med 2014;55(1):88–94.

47. Riola-Parada C, García-Cañamaque L, Pérez-Dueñas V, et al. PET/RM simultánea vs. PET/TC en oncología. Una revisión sistemática. Rev Esp Med Nucl Imagen Mol 2016;35(5):306–12.

48. Boss A, Stegger L, Bisdas S, et al. Feasibility of simultaneous PET/MR imaging in the head and upper neck area. Eur Radiol 2011;21(7):1439–46.

49. Pyatigorskaya N, De Laroche R, Bera G, et al. Are gadolinium-enhanced MR sequences needed in simultaneous 18 F-FDG-PET/MRI for tumor delineation in head and neck cancer? Am J Neuroradiol 2020;41(10):1888–96.

50. Dang H, Chen Y, Zhang Z, et al. Application of integrated positron emission tomography/magnetic resonance imaging in evaluating the prognostic factors of head and neck squamous cell carcinoma with positron emission tomography, diffusion-weighted imaging, dynamic contrast enhancement and. Dentomaxillofac Radiol 2020;49(5):20190488.

51. Hayashi K, Kikuchi M, Imai Y, et al. Clinical value of fused PET/MRI for surgical planning in patients with oral/oropharyngeal carcinoma. Laryngoscope 2020; 130(2):367–74.

52. Heusch P, Sproll C, Buchbender C, et al. Diagnostic accuracy of ultrasound, 18F-FDG-PET/CT, and fused 18F-FDG-PET-MR images with DWI for the detection of cervical lymph node metastases of HNSCC. Clin Oral Investig 2014;18(3):969–78.

53. Platzek I, Beuthien-Baumann B, Schneider M, et al. FDG PET/MR for lymph node staging in head and neck cancer. Eur J Radiol 2014;83(7):1163–8.

54. Partovi S, Kohan A, Vercher-Conejero JL, et al. Qualitative and quantitative performance of 18 F-FDG-PET/MRI versus 18 F-FDG-PET/CT in patients with head and neck cancer. Am J Neuroradiol 2014; 35(10):1970–5.

55. Leibfarth S, Mönnich D, Welz S, et al. A strategy for multimodal deformable image registration to integrate PET/MR into radiotherapy treatment planning. Acta Oncol (Madr) 2013;52(7):1353–9.

56. Rasmussen JH, Nørgaard M, Hansen AE, et al. Feasibility of multiparametric imaging with PET/MR in head and neck squamous cell carcinoma. J Nucl Med 2017;58(1):69–74.

57. Becker M, Varoquaux AD, Combescure C, et al. Local recurrence of squamous cell carcinoma of the head and neck after radio(chemo)therapy: diagnostic performance of FDG-PET/MRI with diffusion-weighted sequences. Eur Radiol 2018;28(2): 651–63.

PET/Computed Tomography
Laryngeal and Hypopharyngeal Cancers

Asha Kandathil, MD[a],*, Rathan M. Subramaniam, MD, PhD, MPH, MBA[b,c]

KEYWORDS

• PET/CT • FDG • HNSCC • Laryngeal cancer • Hypopharyngeal cancer

KEY POINTS

- [18]F FDG-PET/CT has an established role in staging of laryngeal and hypopharyngeal tumors. [18]F FDG-PET/CT has superior detection of locoregional nodal and distant metastases in comparison with CT and MRI.
- Knowledge of laryngeal and hypopharyngeal anatomy and expected pattern of tumor spread aids in tumor staging.
- Biologic aggressiveness of tumors measured with ^{18}F FDG-PET/CT variables, such as maximum standardized uptake value (SUVmax), metabolic tumor volume (MTV), and total lesion glycolysis (TLG), correlates with overall survival.
- [18]F FDG-PET/CT is superior to anatomic imaging in identifying posttreatment local, regional, and distant tumor recurrence.

INTRODUCTION

Laryngeal cancer is the second most common head and neck cancer with an estimated 12,620 new cases and accounting for 3770 deaths in the United States in 2021. About 3000 cancers originate in the hypopharynx.[1] Patients with laryngeal cancer have a 5-year survival rate of 59%. Hypopharyngeal cancer presents late with a 5-year survival rate of 25% to 40%.[2] Most laryngeal and hypopharyngeal tumors are squamous cell carcinomas, occurring in older individuals with a male preponderance. There is a strong association with smoking. Heavy and moderate alcohol use is also a risk factor. Some hypopharyngeal cancers are associated with human papilloma virus infection. Treatment with surgery, radiation therapy, and chemotherapy is aimed at improving survival and preserving function.[3]

LARYNGEAL ANATOMY

The larynx, which is the superior portion of the respiratory tract, articulates superiorly with the hyoid bone and is contiguous inferiorly with the trachea. The laryngeal skeleton is formed by the epiglottis and thyroid cartilages anteriorly and by the cricoid cartilage and three paired arytenoid, corniculate, and cuneiform cartilages posteriorly. There are fat-containing spaces between the mucosa and the supporting skeleton. The aryepiglottic folds, which protect the opening of the laryngeal lumen, extend between the arytenoid cartilage and the lateral margin of the epiglottis. The three anatomic regions of the larynx are the supraglottis, glottis, and subglottis. The supraglottis extends from the tip of the epiglottis to the laryngeal ventricle and includes the epiglottis, false cords, aryepiglottic folds, and vestibule. The false cords, which are infoldings of the membranes, separate the

[a] Department of Radiology, UT Southwestern Medical Center, Dallas, TX, USA; [b] Dean's Office, Otago Medical School, University of Otago, Dunedin, New Zealand; [c] Department of Radiology, Duke University, Durham, NC, USA
* Corresponding author.
E-mail address: Asha.Kandathil@utsouthwestern.edu

PET Clin 17 (2022) 235–248
https://doi.org/10.1016/j.cpet.2021.12.009

vestibule from the ventricle below. The preepiglot-tic and paraglottic spaces are potential sites for tumor spread. The glottis extends for 1 cm below the vestibule and contains the true vocal cords with the anterior and posterior commissure. The subglottis extends from the undersurface of the vocal cords to the inferior margin of the cricoid cartilage. The ventricular complex includes the false cords, true cords, and intervening ventricle. The medial margin of the false cord is formed by the ventricular liga-ment, which extends from the arytenoid to the thy-roid cartilage. The inner margin of the true cord is formed by the vocal ligament, which extends from the vocal process of the arytenoid to the inner side of the thyroid cartilage. On computed tomog-raphy (CT), the false cord is at the level of the aryte-noid cartilage tip and the true cord is at the level of the anteriorly pointing vocal process of the aryte-noid cartilage. About 60% of tumors originate in the glottis, 35% in the supraglottis, and 5% in the subglottis.[1] Tumors that involve the false and true vocal cord are called transglottic tumors.

HYPOPHARYNGEAL ANATOMY

The hypopharynx, which includes the pyriform si-nuses, lateral and posterior hypopharyngeal walls, and postcricoid regions, extends from the oropharynx to the esophagus. The pyriform si-nuses resemble an inverted pyramid, which ex-tends from the pharyngoepiglottic folds to the inferior margin of the cricoid cartilage. It is sepa-rated from the larynx by the aryepiglottic folds. The posterior hypopharyngeal wall is separated from the vertebrae by the retropharyngeal space. The postcricoid region is the anterior wall of the hypopharynx and measures less than 10 mm in anteroposterior diameter (**Figs. 1–3**).

STAGING OF LARYNGEAL AND HYPOPHARYNGEAL TUMORS

The 8th edition of American Joint Committee on Cancer (AJCC) TNM staging system is used to determine disease extent, prognosis, and man-agement.[4] The T stage is based on tumor size, involvement of adjacent structures, and vocal cord mobility. N stage is determined by size and location of involved node and extranodal exten-sion (ENE) into adjacent tissues. M stage refers to distant metastases, best determined by PET with fluorodeoxyglucose F 18 (^{18}F FDG-PET)/CT.

TNM Staging of Laryngeal and Hypopharyngeal Cancer: American Joint Committee on Cancer, Eighth Edition

Primary tumor (T)

TX: Primary tumor cannot be assessed
Tis: Carcinoma in situ
Supraglottis
  T1: Tumor limited to one subsite of supraglot-tis with normal vocal cord mobility
  T2: Tumor invades mucosa of greater than one adjacent subsite of supraglottis or glottis or region outside supraglottis (eg, mucosa of base of tongue, vallecula, medial wall of pyriform sinus) with normal vocal cord mobility
  T3: Tumor limited to larynx with vocal cord fix-ation or invades any of the following: post-cricoid area, preepiglottic space, paraglottic space, or inner cortex of thyroid cartilage
  T4a: Moderately advanced local disease: in-vades through the outer cortex thyroid cartilage or invades tissues beyond the lar-ynx (eg, trachea, soft tissues of neck including deep extrinsic muscle of tongue, strap muscles, thyroid, or esophagus)
  T4b: Very advanced local disease: invades prevertebral space, encases carotid artery, or invades mediastinal structure
Glottis
  T1: Tumor limited to the vocal cords (may involve anterior or posterior commissure) with normal cord mobility
  • *T1a:* Limited to one vocal cord
  • *T1b:* Involves both vocal cords
  T2: Tumor extends to supraglottis and/or sub-glottis and/or with impaired vocal cord mobility
  T3: Tumor limited to the larynx with vocal cord fixation and/or invasion of paraglottic space and/or inner cortex of the thyroid cartilage
  T4a: Moderately advanced local disease: in-vades through the outer cortex of the thy-roid cartilage or invades tissues beyond the larynx (eg, trachea, cricoid cartilage, soft tissues of neck including deep extrinsic muscle of the tongue, strap muscles, thy-roid, or esophagus)
  T4b: Very advanced local disease: invades prevertebral space, encases carotid artery, or invades mediastinal structures
Subglottis
  T1: Tumor limited to subglottis
  T2: Tumor extends to vocal cords with normal or impaired mobility
  T3: Tumor limited to larynx with vocal cord fix-ation or invasion of paraglottic space or in-ner cortex of the thyroid cartilage
  T4a: Moderately advanced local disease: tu-mor invades cricoid or thyroid cartilage or invades tissues beyond the larynx (eg,

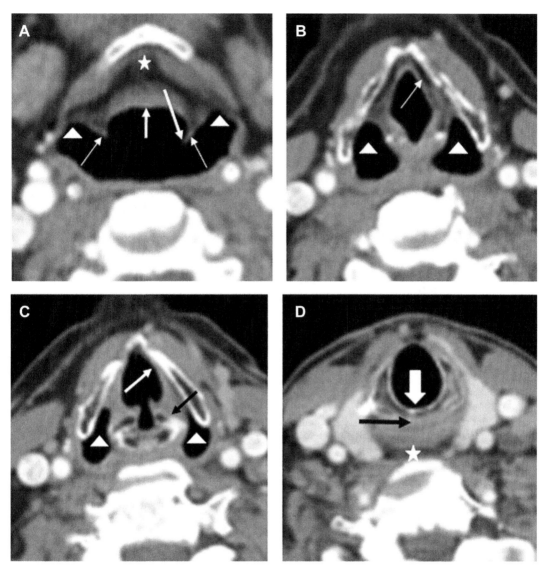

Fig. 1. Normal anatomy of the larynx and hypopharynx on axial CT images. (*A*) The preepiglottic fat (*star*) is anterior to the epiglottis (*white arrows*) and the pyriform sinuses are lateral to the aryepiglottic folds (*triangles*). (*B*) Note the paraglottic fat (*white arrow*) at the level of the false vocal cords. (*C*) At the level of the true vocal cords (*white arrow*) all three cartilages are visualized on one axial image. (*D*) There is normal absence of soft tissue at the level of the cricoid cartilage (*white arrow*). Anterior wall of the hypopharynx is the postcricoid region (*black arrow*) and retropharyngeal space (*star*) is posterior to the hypopharynx.

trachea, soft tissues of neck including deep extrinsic muscles of the tongue, strap muscles, thyroid, or esophagus)

T4b: Very advanced local disease: tumor invades prevertebral space, encases carotid artery, or invades mediastinal structures

Hypopharynx (T)

T1: Tumor limited to one subsite of hypopharynx or ≤2 cm in greatest dimension

T2: Tumor invades greater than one subsite of hypopharynx or an adjacent site or tumor <2 cm but ≤4 cm in greatest dimension without fixation of hemilarynx

T3: Tumor <4 cm in greatest dimension or with fixation of hemilarynx or extension to esophageal mucosa

T4a: Moderately advanced local disease: tumor of any size invading thyroid/cricoid cartilage, hyoid bone, thyroid gland, esophageal muscle, or central compartment soft tissue (prelaryngeal strap muscles and subcutaneous fat)

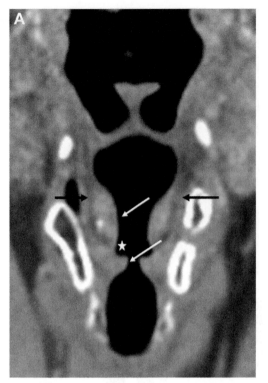

Fig. 2. Normal anatomy of the larynx on coronal CT image. False vocal cord (*top white arrow*) and true vocal cord (*bottom white arrow*) are separated by the ventricle (*star*). Note the paraglottic space (*black arrows*).

> *T4b:* Very advanced local disease: tumor of any size encasing carotid artery or invading prevertebral fascia, or mediastinal structures
>
> Clinical regional lymph node staging (N)
>
> *NX:* Regional lymph nodes cannot be assessed
>
> *N0:* No regional lymph node metastasis
>
> *N1:* Metastasis in a single ipsilateral node ≤3 cm in greatest dimension and no ENE
>
> *N2a:* Single ipsilateral node <3 cm but ≤6 cm and no ENE
>
> *N2b:* Metastases in multiple ipsilateral nodes, all ≤6 cm and no ENE
>
> *N2c:* Metastases in bilateral or contralateral nodes, all ≤6 cm and no ENE
>
> *N3a:* Metastasis in a node <6 cm and no ENE
>
> *N3b:* Metastasis in a node with ENE
>
> Distant metastasis (M)
>
> *M0:* No distant metastasis
>
> *M1:* Distant metastasis

[18]F FDG-PET/computed TOMOGRAPHY EVALUATION OF LARYNGEAL AND HYPOPHARYNGEAL TUMORS

[18]F FDG-PET/CT has a key role in staging, prognostication, and therapeutic response assessment of laryngeal and hypopharyngeal tumors. Leclere and colleagues[5] found that integration of ^{18}F FDG-PET/CT in the initial staging of head and neck squamous cell carcinoma (HNSCC) altered staging in up to 46% of patients, because of changes in lymph node staging in 38.2%, detection of a second primary tumor in 7.3%, or finding occult metastases in 4.5%, allowing better prognostication and optimizing management strategies. A study in 25 patients with histopathologically confirmed HNSCC found no significant differences between ^{18}F FDG-PET/MRI, ^{18}F FDG-PET/CT, and MRI in local tumor staging and identifying recurrent cancer.[6] The 2020 National Comprehensive Cancer Network guidelines state that for initial staging, ^{18}F FDG-PET/CT has superior detection of locoregional nodal and distant metastases in comparison with CT and MRI. According to the guidelines, in patients with high concern for distant metastases ^{18}F FDG-PET/CT may be performed following induction chemotherapy before deciding on definitive local therapy.[18] F FDG-PET/CT is preferred for treatment response assessment following radiotherapy, with a repeat PET/CT scan in 4 to 6 weeks in patients with equivocal results.[7]

ROLE OF ^{18}F FDG-PET/computed TOMOGRAPHY IN STAGING
T Staging

Although PET/CT has high sensitivity in detecting and staging head and neck tumors, because of better spatial and contrast resolution, contrast-enhanced CT or MRI are routinely used to determine tumor size, submucosal spread, cartilage invasion, and involvement of adjacent structures. Knowledge of expected pattern of tumor spread aids in T staging.

Laryngeal tumors: pattern of spread

Glottic tumor Most frequent site of involvement is the anterior portion of the vocal cord. There is often involvement of the anterior commissure and extension into the contralateral vocal cord (**Fig. 4**). There may be invasion of the thyroid cartilage with extralaryngeal spread, extension inferiorly into the anterior subglottic region, or superiorly into the preepiglottic space. Tumors that arise from the posterior aspect of the vocal cord may involve the posterior commissure, postcricoid esophagus, or subglottis. There may be lateral extension into the paraglottic space or extralaryngeal spread through the space between the arytenoid and thyroid cartilage. Even in the absence of cartilage invasion there may be overlap of FDG activity because of blooming artifact. Erosion or lysis of the

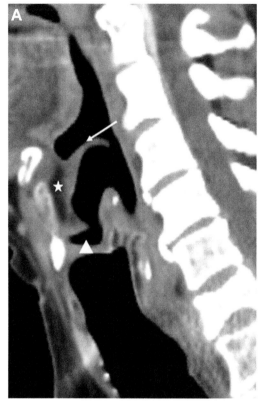

Fig. 3. Normal anatomy of the larynx on sagittal CT image. The preepiglottic fat (*star*) is anterior to the base of the epiglottis (*white arrow*) and superior to the true vocal cord (*triangle*).

cartilage or presence of tumor on the extralaryngeal side of the thyroid or cricoid cartilage are reliable signs of cartilage invasion. T3 tumors extend into the paraglottic and/or preepiglottic space, whereas T4 tumors have extralaryngeal spread (**Fig. 5**).

Supraglottic tumors Epiglottic cancers may spread to the valleculae, tongue base, preepiglottic space, aryepiglottic folds, and false vocal cords. Aryepiglottic fold tumors may involve the paraglottic space and spread to the false and true vocal cords and piriform sinus. Cartilage invasion is rare in supraglottic cancer.

Subglottic tumors Soft tissue thickening between the mucosa and cricoid cartilage is abnormal and suspicious for subglottic tumor. Subglottic tumors may be bilateral or circumferential. There is early invasion of the true vocal cords and cricoid cartilage.

Hypopharyngeal tumors: pattern of spread
Hypopharyngeal tumors have a propensity for submucosal spread. Tumors arising from the medial wall of the pyriform sinus invade the larynx early and extend to the contralateral side. There may be perineural tumor extension. Tumors arising from the lateral wall of the pyriform sinus extend into the paraglottic space, soft tissues of the neck, and invade the posterior aspect of the thyroid cartilage.

Posterior hypopharyngeal wall tumors can grow along the posterior pharyngeal wall superiorly up to the nasopharynx and inferiorly to the cervical esophagus. There may be extension posteriorly to involve the prevertebral muscles with loss of the prevertebral fat planes (**Fig. 6**).

Postcricoid tumors tend to invade the posterior aspect of the larynx and pyriform sinuses. There may be inferior extension into the esophagus or trachea.

Pitfalls in T staging by ¹⁸F FDG-PET/computed tomography
Physiologic FDG uptake in lymphoid tissue and muscles may mimic tumor infiltration. Asymmetric

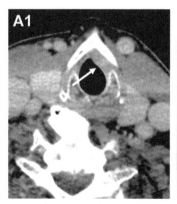

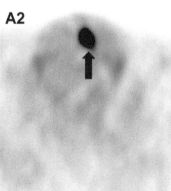

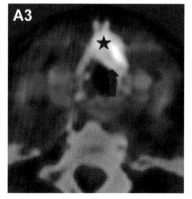

Fig. 4. A 54-year-old man with laryngeal cancer. FDG-avid thickening of the left vocal cord (*arrow*) and anterior commissure (*star*).

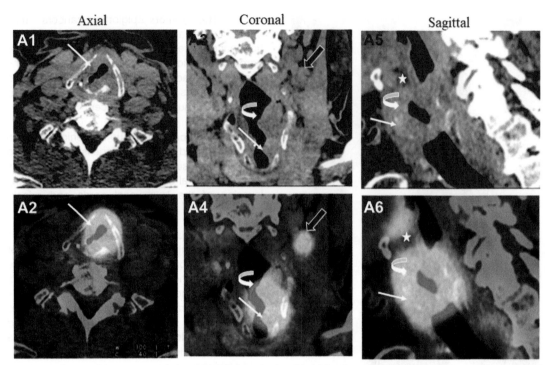

Fig. 5. A 72-year-old woman with laryngeal cancer. FDG-avid thickening of the left and right vocal cords with involvement of the anterior and posterior commissures (*White arrow*). There is involvement of the supraglottis (*curved arrows*) with extension into the preepiglottic space (*star*). FDG-avid left level 2 metastatic node (*black arrow*).

lymphoid tissue uptake and focal rather than diffuse uptake in muscle is concerning for tumor involvement. Physiologic FDG uptake in the crico-pharyngeus muscle can mimic postcricoid tumor; however, adjacent fat planes are preserved. If the patient was talking during FDG uptake phase there may be intense uptake in the laryngeal musculature. Unilateral vocal cord paralysis with FDG uptake in the contralateral mobile vocal cord can be mistaken for malignancy. Perineural tumor spread may be lower than the resolution of PET and intracranial extension may be masked by physiologic FDG uptake by brain parenchyma. FDG uptake in brown fat in the neck can impair

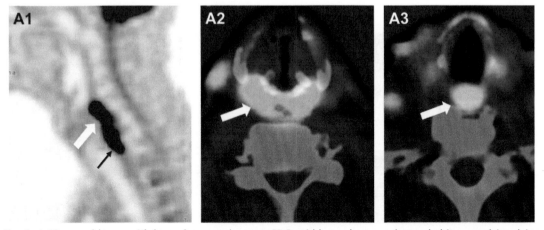

Fig. 6. A 60-year-old man with hypopharyngeal cancer. FDG-avid hypopharyngeal mass (*white arrow*) involving the upper cervical esophagus (*black arrow*).

detection of FDG-avid nodes. Ensuring that the patient is warm and not talking or chewing during FDG injection and uptake minimizes physiologic uptake.

N Staging

The AJCC staging criteria is similar for laryngeal and hypopharyngeal cancer. Direction of nodal metastases depends on lymphatic drainage of the involved region, tumor size and extent, and prior surgery. Contralateral node involvement is possible in tumors close to midline. Laryngeal and hypopharyngeal tumors rarely metastasize to level 1 or 5 nodes.

Laryngeal cancer
Glottic tumors confined to the vocal cord have decreased propensity for lymphatic spread. Nodal metastases is more common after breach of the anterior commissure or involvement of the supraglottis or subglottis. Cervical node level 3 is most commonly involved with levels 2, 4, and 6 involved to a lesser extent. Prelaryngeal (delphian) lymph node may be involved.

Supraglottic tumors metastasize to level 2 and 3 nodes and have a propensity for contralateral involvement. Tumors involving the preepiglottic fat metastasize early to bilateral level 2 to 4 nodes.

Subglottic tumors metastasize to level 4 and level 3 nodes.

Hypopharyngeal cancer
Hypopharyngeal tumors have a propensity for early nodal metastases. Pyriform sinus tumors metastasize to level 2, 3, and 4 nodes. Tumors involving the medial wall of the pyriform sinus can metastasize to contralateral nodes. Postcricoid tumors drain to level 3, 4, and 6 nodes. Posterior hypopharyngeal tumors metastasize to retropharyngeal nodes and secondarily to level 3, 4, and 6 nodes (**Fig. 7**).

Nodal staging impacts the treatment and prognosis of patients with laryngeal and hypopharyngeal cancers. On PET/CT, features suggestive of metastases include increased FDG avidity greater than neck blood pool,[8] increased size with short axis diameter more than 10 mm, round shape, necrosis, and ill-defined margins suggestive of ENE. Retropharyngeal nodes greater than or equal to 6 mm in short axis diameter are considered to be enlarged.[9]

In a meta-analysis of 32 studies ^{18}F FDG-PET/CT had sensitivity and specificity of 80% and 86%, respectively, in detecting lymph node metastases in patients with HNSCC as compared with 75% and 79%, respectively, for CT and MRI.[10] False-positive FDG uptake can occur in reactive nodes. There may be falsely decreased FDG uptake in small or necrotic nodes with metastases. Metabolic activity in metastatic nodes adjacent to an intensely FDG-avid adjacent primary tumor may be obscured. Extracapsular tumor extension, an important predictor of recurrence, upstages nodal stage in the eighth edition of the TNM Classification for head and neck tumors. In a study on 94 patients with HNSCC. Toya and colleagues[11] found that maximum standardized uptake value (SUVmax) of greater than or equal to 3.0 provided appropriate diagnostic value in identifying ENE.

M Staging

Most common site for distant metastases from head and neck cancer is the lungs, followed by liver, bone, and skin. Patients with head and neck cancer also have increased risk for second primary tumors in the head and neck or lungs. Kim and colleagues[12] report sensitivity of 97.5%,

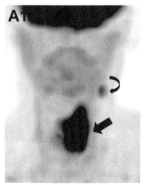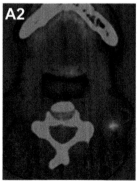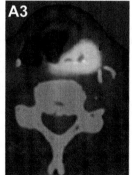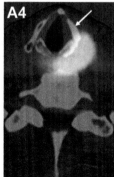

Fig. 7. A 48-year-old man with hypopharyngeal cancer. FDG-avid mass involving the left pyriform sinus with extension inferiorly into the left paraglottic space (*black arrow*), lateral to the thyroid cartilage (*white arrow*). FDG-avid left level 2 metastatic node (*curved arrow*).

a specificity of 92.6%, a positive predictive value of 62.9%, and a negative predictive value of 99.7% for ^{18}F FDG-PET/CT in detecting second primary cancers and distant metastases in patients with HNSCC. National Comprehensive Cancer Network guidelines recommend ^{18}F FDG-PET/CT scan for evaluation of distant metastases with directed CT or MRI to evaluate specific areas of concern, such as lung or bone.

ROLE OF ^{18}F FDG-PET/computed TOMOGRAPHY IN PROGNOSTICATION

Biologic aggressiveness of tumors measured with ^{18}F FDG-PET/CT variables, such as SUVmax, metabolic tumor volume (MTV), and total lesion glycolysis (TLG), correlates with overall survival in patients with head and neck cancer.[13] Romesser and colleagues[14] found that in patients with HNSCC treated with intensity-modulated radiotherapy SUVmax correlated significantly with AJCC stage, with stage 4 tumors having a higher SUVmax than stage 1 to 3 tumors. In a study by Kitajima and colleagues,[15] patients with laryngeal cancer with high SUVmax ($\geq$4) in nodal metastases had a significantly lower progression-free survival rate. MTV derived from pretreatment ^{18}F FDG-PET/CT has been found to be an independent predictor of locoregional disease control and overall survival in patients with locoregionally advanced squamous cell carcinoma of the larynx and hypopharynx.[16] Suzuki and colleagues[17] found that TLG greater than or equal to 5.4 correlated significantly with shorter overall survival in patients with laryngopharyngeal squamous cell carcinoma. In patients with hypopharyngeal squamous cell carcinoma, SUVmax greater than or equal to 28.5 and TLG greater than or equal to 42 was found to be associated with shorter overall survival time.[18] Radiomic features extracted from pretreatment ^{18}F FDG-PET/CT, such as MTV, grey-level zone length matrix, and small-zone low grey-level emphasis, show promise in predicting early disease progression in patients with locally advanced squamous cell carcinoma of the larynx and hypopharynx.[19]

ROLE OF ^{18}F FDG-PET/computed TOMOGRAPHY IN TREATMENT PLANNING

In radiotherapy planning use of ^{18}F FDG-PET/CT has been found to result in smaller primary tumor volumes in comparison with use of CT. There is, however, no significant difference between the two modalities in contouring of nodes.[20] In a study by Daisne and colleagues,[21] tumor volume measured on ^{18}F FDG-PET/CT in patients with laryngeal tumors correlated best with pathologic tumor volume in nine patients who underwent laryngectomy. MTV measured on ^{18}F-FDG-PET has been found to be closely associated with pathologic tumor volume and TLG was found to be associated with tumor thickness and depth of invasion.[18]

ROLE OF ^{18}F FDG-PET/computed TOMOGRAPHY IN POSTTREATMENT RESPONSE ASSESSMENT

Depending on the tumor stage laryngeal and hypopharyngeal tumors may be treated with surgery, chemotherapy, radiotherapy, or definitive chemoradiation with organ preservation. Patients with laryngeal and hypopharyngeal tumors may have locoregional recurrence or distant metastases. If local tumor recurrence is detected early it could potentially be retreated with local therapy. [18]F FDG-PET/CT is superior to anatomic imaging in identifying posttreatment local, regional, and distant tumor recurrence. To minimize false-positive results caused by inflammation, ^{18}F FDG-PET/CT should be performed 12 weeks postchemoradiotherapy (**Fig. 8**).

Patients with laryngeal cancer who had ^{18}F FDG-PET/CT surveillance during the first 6 months were found to have better survival as compared with those who had CT surveillance.[22] There are several interpretative criteria for treatment response assessment, such as the Neck Imaging Reporting and Data Systems, Porceddu, Hopkins, and Deauville scoring systems, which rely on visual assessment of FDG uptake in the tumor or metastatic node relative to adjacent tissues and liver.[23] The five-point Hopkins criteria has 91.1% negative predictive value and 86.9% accuracy in therapeutic response assessment.[8] Hopkins criteria for posttherapy assessment of tumor or metastatic node in PET/CT is as follows:

1. Minimal uptake (<internal jugular vein): complete metabolic response
2. Minimal uptake (>internal jugular vein but <liver): probably complete metabolic response
3. Diffuse uptake (>internal jugular vein and liver): probably postradiation inflammation
4. Moderate focal uptake (>liver): probably persistent tumor
5. Intense focal uptake (>liver): persistent tumor

In patients suspected of locoregional recurrence following laryngectomy with or without adjuvant radiotherapy, ^{18}F FDG-PET/CT has been found to have sensitivity, specificity, and accuracy of 100%, 87.5%, and 91.6%, respectively, for local

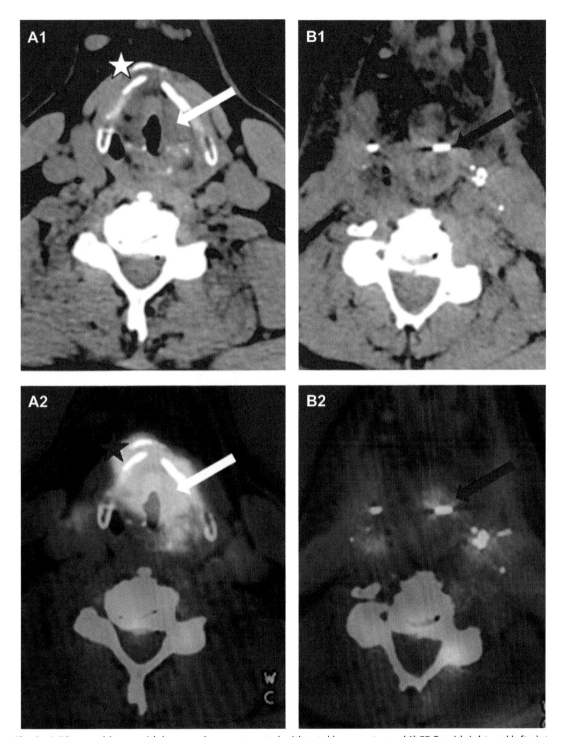

Fig. 8. A 56-year-old man with laryngeal cancer, treated with total laryngectomy. (*A*) FDG-avid right and left glottic mass (*white arrow*) involving the anterior commissure and thyroid cartilage (*star*). (*B*) No FDG-avid residual tumor in the laryngectomy bed (*black arrow*).

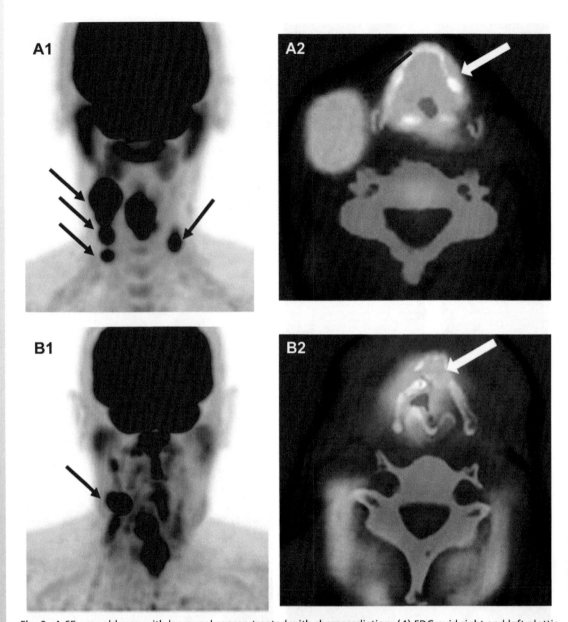

Fig. 9. A 65-year-old man with laryngeal cancer, treated with chemoradiation. (*A*) FDG-avid right and left glottic mass (*white arrow*) involving the anterior commissure. Bilateral FDG-avid metastatic cervical nodes (*black arrows*). (*B*) Partial metabolic response with residual FDG-avid laryngeal mass (*white arrow*) and residual FDG-avid right cervical node (*black arrow*).

tumor recurrence and sensitivity, specificity, and accuracy of 100%, 90%, and 95.4%, respectively, for detection of nodal recurrence.[24] In a meta-analysis of three studies evaluating local recurrence of laryngeal cancer detected by PET/CT following chemoradiotherapy the sensitivity of ^{18}F FDG-PET/CT performed 2 to 12 months after treatment ranged from 33% to 75%, specificity from 53% to 86%, positive predictive value from

40% to 67%, and negative predictive value from 73% to 86%.[25] The RELAPS multicenter randomized trial by de Bree and colleagues[26] showed that evaluation by ^{18}F FDG-PET/CT following radiotherapy for laryngeal cancer lowers the need for direct laryngoscopies under general anesthesia by 50%.

In patients undergoing salvage treatment following recurrence of laryngohypopharyngeal

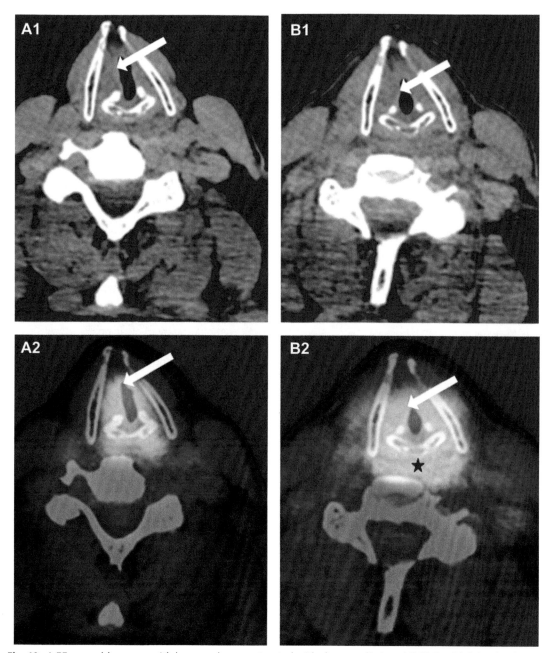

Fig. 10. A 55-year-old woman with laryngeal cancer, treated with chemoradiation. (*A*) FDG-avid right glottic mass (*white arrow*). (*B*) Residual FDG-avid mass in the glottis. Note increased FDG uptake in the hypopharynx (*star*) caused by postradiation inflammation.

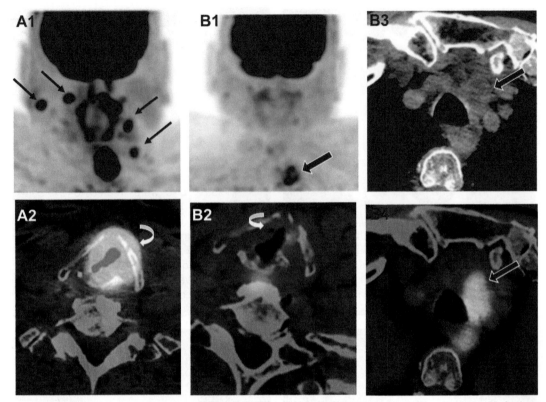

Fig. 11. A 70-year-old man with laryngeal cancer, treated with chemoradiation. (*A*) FDG-avid right and left glottic mass with extralaryngeal extension (*curved arrow*) and bilateral metastatic nodes (*black arrows*). (*B*) Complete metabolic response of laryngeal mass and nodes. New FDG-avid necrotic metastatic node with extranodal extension (*black arrow*) in the left superior mediastinum.

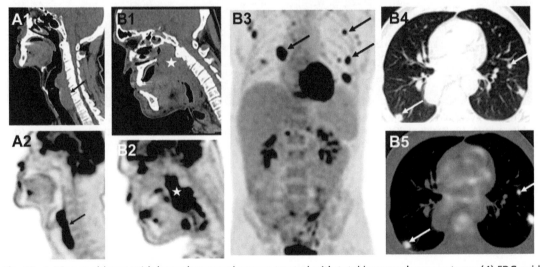

Fig. 12. A 56-year-old man with hypopharyngeal cancer, treated with total laryngopharyngectomy. (*A*) FDG-avid hypopharyngeal mass (*arrow*) extending into the cervical esophagus. (*B*) Recurrent FDG-avid mass in the nasopharynx (*star*) with multiple FDG-avid lung metastases (*arrows*).

squamous cell carcinoma, PET parameters of SUVmax (>4.0), MTV (>6.5 mL), and TLG (>17.1 g) in recurrent tumors were significantly associated with poor progression-free survival and poor overall survival (**Figs. 9–12**).[27]

SUMMARY

^{18}F FDG-PET/CT has an established role in staging, prognostication, and therapeutic response assessment of laryngeal and hypopharyngeal tumors. Knowledge of cross-sectional laryngeal and hypopharyngeal anatomy, expected patterns of tumor spread and awareness of physiologic FDG uptake in head and neck structures is essential for accurate TNM staging and therapy response assessment of laryngeal and hypopharyngeal cancers.

CLINICS CARE POINTS

- ^{18}F FDG-PET/CT is an integral part of clinical staging of patients with laryngeal and hypopharyngeal cancer, optimizing management strategies.
- ^{18}F FDG-PET/CT is the standard of care in identifying posttreatment local, regional, and distant tumor recurrence.

DISCLOSURE

The authors have nothing to disclose.

REFERENCES

1. Available at: https://www.cancer.org/cancer/laryngeal-and-hypopharyngeal-cancer/about/key-statistics.html. Accessed January 18, 2022.
2. Eckel HE, Bradley PJ. Natural history of treated and untreated hypopharyngeal cancer. Adv Otorhinolaryngol 2019;83:27–34.
3. Siegel RL, Miller KD, Jemal A. Cancer statistics, 2020. CA Cancer J Clin 2020;70(1):7–30.
4. Amin MB, Greene FL, Edge SB, et al. The Eighth Edition AJCC Cancer Staging Manual: continuing to build a bridge from a population-based to a more "personalized" approach to cancer staging. CA Cancer J Clin 2017;67(2):93–9.
5. Leclere JC, Delcroix O, Rousset J, et al. Integration of 18-FDG PET/CT in the initial work-up to stage head and neck cancer: prognostic significance and impact on therapeutic decision making. Front Med (Lausanne) 2020;7:273.
6. Schaarschmidt BM, Heusch P, Buchbender C, et al. Locoregional tumour evaluation of squamous cell carcinoma in the head and neck area: a comparison between MRI, PET/CT and integrated PET/MRI. Eur J Nucl Med Mol Imaging 2016;43(1):92–102.
7. Pfister DG, Spencer S, Adelstein D, et al. Head and Neck Cancers, Version 2.2020, NCCN clinical practice guidelines in oncology. J Natl Compr Canc Netw 2020;18(7):873–98.
8. Marcus C, Ciarallo A, Tahari AK, et al. Head and neck PET/CT: therapy response interpretation criteria (Hopkins Criteria)-interreader reliability, accuracy, and survival outcomes. J Nucl Med 2014;55(9):1411–6.
9. Zhang GY, Liu LZ, Wei WH, et al. Radiologic criteria of retropharyngeal lymph node metastasis in nasopharyngeal carcinoma treated with radiation therapy. Radiology 2010;255(2):605–12.
10. Kyzas PA, Evangelou E, Denaxa-Kyza D, et al. 18F-fluorodeoxyglucose positron emission tomography to evaluate cervical node metastases in patients with head and neck squamous cell carcinoma: a meta-analysis. J Natl Cancer Inst 2008;100(10):712–20.
11. Toya R, Saito T, Matsuyama T, et al. Diagnostic value of FDG-PET/CT for the identification of extranodal extension in patients with head and neck squamous cell carcinoma. Anticancer Res 2020;40(4):2073–7.
12. Kim SY, Roh JL, Yeo NK, et al. Combined 18F-fluorodeoxyglucose-positron emission tomography and computed tomography as a primary screening method for detecting second primary cancers and distant metastases in patients with head and neck cancer. Ann Oncol 2007;18(10):1698–703.
13. Pak K, Cheon GJ, Nam HY, et al. Prognostic value of metabolic tumor volume and total lesion glycolysis in head and neck cancer: a systematic review and meta-analysis. J Nucl Med 2014;55(6):884–90.
14. Romesser PB, Qureshi MM, Shah BA, et al. Superior prognostic utility of gross and metabolic tumor volume compared to standardized uptake value using PET/CT in head and neck squamous cell carcinoma patients treated with intensity-modulated radiotherapy. Ann Nucl Med 2012;26(7):527–34.
15. Kitajima K, Suenaga Y, Kanda T, et al. Prognostic value of FDG PET imaging in patients with laryngeal cancer. PLoS One 2014;9(5):e96999.
16. Park GC, Kim JS, Roh JL, et al. Prognostic value of metabolic tumor volume measured by 18F-FDG PET/CT in advanced-stage squamous cell carcinoma of the larynx and hypopharynx. Ann Oncol 2013;24(1):208–14.
17. Suzuki H, Tamaki T, Nishio M, et al. Total lesion glycolysis on FDG-PET/CT before salvage surgery predicts survival in laryngeal or pharyngeal cancer. Oncotarget 2018;9(27):19115–22.
18. Suzuki H, Nishio M, Nakanishi H, et al. Impact of total lesion glycolysis measured by (18)F-FDG-PET/CT on overall survival and distant metastasis in

hypopharyngeal cancer. Oncol Lett 2016;12(2): 1493–500.

19. Zhong J, Frood R, Brown P, et al. Machine learning-based FDG PET-CT radiomics for outcome prediction in larynx and hypopharynx squamous cell carcinoma. Clin Radiol 2021;76(1):78.e9-17.

20. Cacicedo J, Navarro A, Del Hoyo O, et al. Role of fluorine-18 fluorodeoxyglucose PET/CT in head and neck oncology: the point of view of the radiation oncologist. Br J Radiol 2016;89(1067):20160217.

21. Daisne JF, Duprez T, Weynand B, et al. Tumor volume in pharyngolaryngeal squamous cell carcinoma: comparison at CT, MR imaging, and FDG PET and validation with surgical specimen. Radiology 2004;233(1):93–100.

22. Karam RMAS. Surveillance imaging of laryngeal cancer: does FDG PET/CT impact survival? J Nucl Med 2020;61:1291.

23. Zhong J, Sundersingh M, Dyker K, et al. Post-treatment FDG PET-CT in head and neck carcinoma: comparative analysis of 4 qualitative interpretative criteria in a large patient cohort. Sci Rep 2020; 10(1):4086.

24. Allegra ESV, De Natale M, Marino N, et al. Use of PET/CT to detect local and regional laryngeal cancer recurrence after surgery. Rep Med Imaging 2017;10:31–6.

25. Seebauer CT, Hackenberg B, Grosse J, et al. Routine restaging after primary non-surgical treatment of laryngeal squamous cell carcinoma: a review. Strahlenther Onkol 2021;197(3):167–76.

26. de Bree R, van der Putten L, van Tinteren H, et al. Effectiveness of an (18)F-FDG-PET based strategy to optimize the diagnostic trajectory of suspected recurrent laryngeal carcinoma after radiotherapy: the RELAPS multicenter randomized trial. Radiother Oncol 2016;118(2):251–6.

27. Lee JR, Almuhaimid TM, Roh JL, et al. Prognostic value of (18) F-FDG PET/CT parameters in patients who undergo salvage treatments for recurrent squamous cell carcinoma of the larynx and hypopharynx. J Surg Oncol 2018;118(4):644–50.

18F-fluorodeoxyglucose PET/Computed Tomography
Head and Neck Salivary Gland Tumors

Stephen M. Broski, MD[a],*, Derek R. Johnson, MD[a,b], Annie T. Packard, MD[a], Christopher H. Hunt, MD[a,b]

KEYWORDS

- PET/CT • Salivary gland tumor • Staging • Prognostic

KEY POINTS

- 18F-fluorodeoxyglucose (FDG) PET/computed tomography (CT) is beneficial in staging and restaging salivary gland tumors, by accurately delineating locoregional and distant metastatic disease.
- Numerous studies have demonstrated that the information provided by PET/CT has important prognostic implications for salivary gland malignancies.
- FDG PET/CT has not been shown to be helpful in differentiating benign and malignant salivary gland tumors.
- Several investigational non-FDG PET radiotracers have utility for evaluating salivary gland tumors and point to a potential role for targeted radiotherapy in treatment of salivary gland cancer.

INTRODUCTION

Salivary gland tumors (SGTs) are a heterogenous group of neoplasms arising from the 3 pairs of major salivary glands (parotid, submandibular, and sublingual) or the numerous minor salivary glands located throughout the oral cavity. The most recent version of the World Health Organization (WHO) classification of head and neck tumors recognizes more than 30 distinct benign and malignant salivary gland neoplasms,[1] as shown in **Box 1.**

Overall, the most common SGT is pleomorphic adenoma, a benign tumor that accounts for approximately half of all salivary tumors. Among the numerous malignant salivary cancer types, the 2 most common are adenoid cystic carcinoma (ACC) and mucoepidermoid carcinoma (MEC). The parotid gland is by far the most common site of major salivary gland neoplasm, representing approximately 80% of these tumors. Only approximately a quarter of parotid neoplasms, however, are malignant. Conversely, approximately half of submandibular gland tumors and most sublingual gland and minor SGTs are malignant.

SGTs are relatively rare, representing only 6% to 8% of head and neck neoplasms. The incidence of major salivary gland cancer (SGC), however, has increased over time, from 10.4 cases per 100,000 in 1973 to 16 per 100,000 in 2009,[2] with increasing incidence of both parotid and extraparotid tumors. The reason for this trend is unknown, because there are few known risk factors for SGC beyond patient age and radiation exposure.[3,4] Smoking is strongly associated with risk of Warthin tumor,[5,6] a benign neoplasm, but not with risk of salivary malignancy. SGTs, with the exception of ACC and acinic cell carcinoma, are more common in men, and men also are more likely to present with regional or distant spread of disease.[7]

a Department of Radiology, Mayo Clinic, Rochester, MN, USA; b Department of Neurology, Mayo Clinic, Rochester, MN, USA
* Corresponding author. Mayo Clinic, Charlton Building North, First Floor, 200 First Street Southwest, Rochester, MN 55905.
E-mail address: Broski.stephen@mayo.edu

PET Clin 17 (2022) 249–263
https://doi.org/10.1016/j.cpet.2021.12.002

Box 1
World Health Organization classification of salivary gland tumors

Benign

- Pleomorphic adenoma
- Myoepithelioma
- Basal cell adenoma
- Warthin tumor
- Oncocytoma
- Lymphadenoma
- Cystadenoma
- Sialadenoma papilliferum
- Ductal papillomas
- Sebaceous adenoma
- Canalicular adenoma and other ductal adenomas

Malignant

- Mucoepidermoid carcinoma
- Adenoid cystic carcinoma
- Acinic cell carcinoma
- Polymorphous adenocarcinoma
- Clear cell carcinoma
- Basal cell adenocarcinoma
- Intraductal carcinoma
- Adenocarcinoma, not otherwise specified
- Salivary duct carcinoma
- Myoepithelial carcinoma
- Epithelial-myoepithelial carcinoma
- Carcinoma ex pleomorphic adenoma
- Secretory carcinoma
- Sebaceous adenocarcinoma
- Carcinosarcoma
- Poorly differentiated carcinoma
- Lymphoepithelial carcinoma
- Squamous cell carcinoma
- Oncocytic carcinoma
- Sialoblastoma

Data from El-Naggar AK, Chan JKC, Grandis JR, Takata T, Slootweg PJ. *WHO Classification of Head and Neck Tumours.* International Agency for Research on Cancer; 2017.

CLINICAL PRESENTATION AND EVALUATION

Most major SGTs present clinically as painless masses. Malignant major SGTs also are more likely than benign tumors to cause symptoms related to involvement of adjacent structures, such as facial weakness, due to invasion of the segment of the facial nerve passing through the parotid gland. Major SGTs also commonly are discovered incidentally on imaging obtained for other reasons. In 1 large series, more than 10% of parotidectomies performed from 2004 to 2013 were in patients with incidentally discovered lesions.[8] The clinical presentation of minor SGTs is more variable due to their widespread anatomic distribution throughout the oral cavity and aerodigestive tract. Tumors within the oral cavity may present relatively early as painless masses or mucosal ulceration, whereas tumors at other sites, such as the nasal cavity, may become large and invasive prior to symptomatic presentation.

The initial evaluation of a patient with an SGT should include a history and physical examination aimed at identifying non-neoplastic etiologies, such as inflammatory or obstructive processes, as well as evaluating the patient for signs and symptoms worrisome for malignancy, such as facial weakness or numbness. In the absence of an identifiable non-neoplastic etiology, a discrete parotid or submandibular gland mass should prompt consideration of ultrasound-guided fine-needle aspiration biopsy, because both benign and malignant tumors are relatively common at these locations and the distinction has significant implications for treatment planning. If biopsy demonstrates a benign lesion, it may be observed or resected, whereas neck dissection may be offered in cases of malignant tumors. Interpretation of biopsy results must be informed, however, by the entirety of the clinical picture, because false-negative biopsy results can occur in patients with malignant lesions.[9] Because sublingual gland tumors are likely to be malignant, surgical removal is the treatment of choice, with extent of surgery depending on tumor size and clinical factors.[10]

Although minor SGTs are diverse in location, pathology, and clinical presentation, the palate is the most common location, and approximately half of palatal minor SGTs are malignant. Both benign and malignant palatal tumors may present with a painless mass or mucosal ulceration, whereas pain is highly worrisome for malignancy.[11] Given the numerous types of minor salivary gland malignancy, incisional biopsy rather than needle biopsy is preferred to allow for histopathologic diagnosis.

RELEVANT ANATOMY
Major Versus Minor Salivary Gland

The salivary glands of the head and neck typically are divided into 2 major subgroups: major and minor. The major salivary glands are readily apparent on most imaging modalities and consist of the paired bilateral parotid, submandibular, and sublingual glands[12] (**Fig. 1**). The largest of the major salivary glands, the parotid gland, is unique in that it is encapsulated, and, as a result, can contain lymph nodes, which can be mistaken for other masses/tumors.[13] The parotid gland, both surgically and from an imaging point of view, often is divided into superficial and deep lobes. The surgical landmark for division of the superficial and deep lobes is the facial nerve, which typically is not evident as it courses through the gland on PET/CT. The retromandibular vein, however, is a reasonable surrogate for the location of the facial nerve and can help delineate the superficial from the deep parotid gland. Approximately 20% of patients also have an accessory parotid gland, which is located anterior to the main parotid gland and superficial to the masseter muscle.[12,14] The normal minor salivary glands typically are not seen with conventional imaging. Although minor salivary glands are widely dispersed deep to the mucosa of the oral cavity, there are numerous additional minor salivary glands distributed throughout the aerodigestive tract, including the sinonasal cavity, pharynx, trachea, and bronchi.

Relevant Anatomic Spaces of the Head and Neck

Lymphatic drainage from the major salivary glands typically is to level I and level II cervical lymph node stations, and these should be scrutinized when imaging a salivary gland malignancy. Although the typical anatomic depiction of cervical nodal stations is well recognized by most radiologists, in reality this depiction, drawn from the perspective of the surgeon or anatomist, can be challenging to quickly translate into cross-sectional imaging. For the purpose of scrutinizing and describing level I and level II nodes, an axial CT image through the floor of the mouth above the level of the hyoid bone typically can provide the required anatomic boundaries for these nodal stations[15] (**Fig. 2**).

The parotid glands drain to both intraglandular and extraglandular lymph nodes, which in turn drain through infra-auricular and upper jugular (level II) lymph nodes. Intraglandular lymph nodes are unique to the parotids and are not found in other major salivary glands. The submandibular glands drain into local nodes, collectively known as submandibular or level IB nodes, although some authorities further divide these into 5 or 6 subsets. The sublingual glands drain into a group of in-transit lymph nodes, referred to as the lingual nodes, which are inconsistently present, and then into the submental (level IA) or submandibular (IB) nodes. Drainage of accessory salivary glands is highly variable, depending on their location. None of the major salivary glands drains into lymph node groups exclusive to the glands, and all the previously noted nodal groups, including the intraglandular lymph nodes of the parotid, may be sites of metastasis by nonsalivary tumors.

ROLE OF PET/COMPUTED TOMOGRAPHY IN HEAD AND NECK SALIVARY GLAND TUMORS
^{18}F-fluorodeoxyglucose PET/Computed Tomography in Differentiating Benign and Malignant Salivary Gland Tumors

Malignant SGTs may be difficult to diagnose prior to surgical resection or biopsy, and discriminating benign from malignant lesions with imaging is problematic. Numerous studies have evaluated the role of ^{18}F-fluorodeoxyglucose (FDG) PET or PET/CT in differentiating benign and malignant SGTs, particularly of the parotid glands, with conflicting results.[16–22] Some investigators have suggested that benign and malignant tumors differ significantly in the degree of FDG uptake[18] or in derived parameters, such as metabolic heterogeneity factor.[16,23] Park and colleagues[21] found that the presence of heterogeneous uptake on

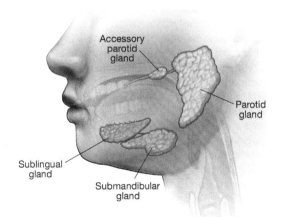

Fig. 1. Illustration depicting the locations of the major salivary glands. (Used with permission of Mayo Foundation for Medical Education and Research, all rights reserved.)

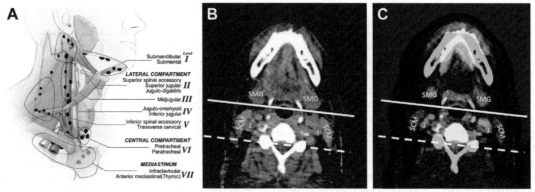

Fig. 2. The traditional image of cervical nodal stations is useful to fully appreciate the anatomic boundaries (*A*) (used with permission of Mayo Foundation for Medical Education and Research, all rights reserved) but can be challenging to quickly translate for use in cross-sectional imaging. Because most SGTs spread to levels I, IIA, and IIB cervical nodal stations, the easiest way to delineate these boundaries is on a single axial slice through the floor of the mouth in the suprahyoid neck (*B*, *C*). Any nodes anterior to the solid white line drawn through the posterior margin of the submandibular gland (SMG) are level I nodes. Any nodes posterior to the posterior border of the SMG but anterior to the posterior border of the sternocleidomastoid (SCM) (*broken white line*) are level II cervical nodes. Level II nodes can be further subdivided into IIA and IIB by the jugular vein (J). Level II nodes anterior to the jugular vein or touching the jugular vein are IIA, with all others being IIB.

PET and ill-defined margins on CT were more likely in malignant FDG-avid parotid lesions and that these combined FDG PET/CT features had better accuracy than PET- or CT-only criteria. Other studies have reported, however, that PET/CT is not able to reliably distinguish between benign parotid tumors, malignant parotid tumors, and metastatic disease to the parotid gland.[24,25] This mainly is because of overlapping metabolic activity between benign and malignant tumor types; specifically, benign lesions, such as Warthin tumor (**Fig. 3**) and pleomorphic adenoma (**Fig. 4**), may show intense FDG uptake in ranges indistinguishable from high-grade, malignant SGTs.[26] In several studies, Warthin tumors represented a significant proportion of false-positive results for malignancy on PET.[25] To complicate matters further, some low-grade malignant histologies, such as acinic cell carcinoma, clear cell carcinoma, and low-grade MEC and ACC (**Fig. 5**), demonstrate lower-level FDG uptake.[17]

Relatively little has been published regarding the role of PET in nonparotid SGTs, likely related to their rarity. In a study evaluating the utility of PET/CT in the evaluation of submandibular and sublingual gland tumors, there was no significant difference in maximum standardized uptake value (SUVmax) values between benign and malignant tumors.[27] Although the positive predictive value of high FDG uptake for malignancy was good, at 84.6%, the negative predictive value of low uptake was poor, at 20%. Dual-time-point PET/CT imaging also has not been found useful in differentiating benign and malignant SGTs, because benign

SGTs may exhibit high uptake, which increases in the delayed phase.[28] Overall, PET/CT has not been found particularly helpful in differentiating benign and malignant SGTs and therefore has not become part of the standard of care or displaced fine-needle biopsy for this purpose.

^{18}F-fluorodeoxyglucose PET/Computed Tomography in Staging Salivary Gland Cancer

Staging of salivary gland malignancy uses the standard TNM (primary tumor [T], regional lymph nodes [N], and distant metastasis [M]) classification system. **Box 2** displays the eighth edition of the major SGT staging schema from the American Joint Committee on Cancer (AJCC).[29] Imaging plays a significant role in salivary malignancy staging, although the role of PET imaging is variable.

Factors that have an impact on the T stage category of the TNM classification, such as tumor size, extraparenchymal extension, and invasion of adjacent structures, generally are assessed with contrast-enhanced CT or MR imaging of the head and neck rather than by PET. Although PET imaging can be helpful with certain aspects of T staging, such as identification of perineural spread (PNS) along the facial nerve from a parotid tumor, the technique currently has a secondary role. In the future, simultaneous PET/MR imaging combining the anatomic detail of MR imaging and the physiologic information of PET may bring nuclear imaging to the forefront.

With respect to evaluation of regional lymph nodes to determine the N category of staging,

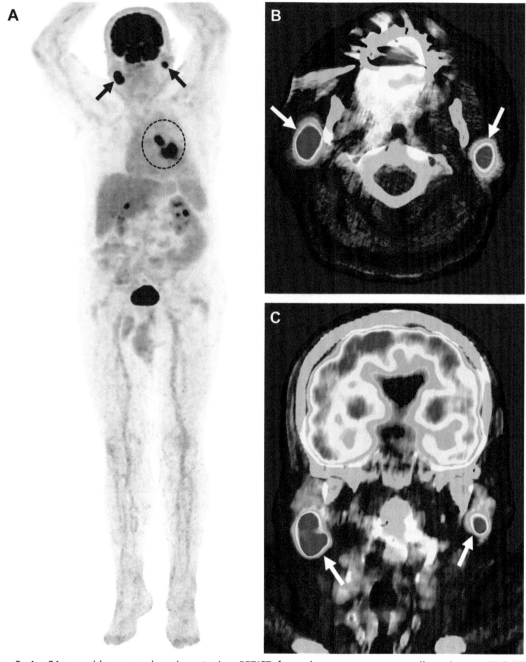

Fig. 3. An 84-year-old man undergoing staging PET/CT for pulmonary squamous cell carcinoma. FDG PET maximum intensity projection image (A) demonstrates an FDG-avid left lower lobe mass with metastatic left hilar lymphadenopathy (dashed circle) and bilateral FDG-avid parotid masses (arrows). Axial (B) and coronal fused PET/CT (C) images demonstrate FDG-avid bilateral parotid masses (arrows), with SUVmax 17.5 on the right and SUVmax 12.8 on the left. Subsequent biopsy confirmed bilateral Warthin tumors.

PET imaging has proved very useful (Figs. 6 and 7). Studies suggest that PET/CT is superior to CT or MR imaging in identification of lymph node metastases from SGTs.[27,30] For example, Westergaard-Nielsen and colleagues[30] prospectively examined the impact of staging FDG PET/CT in suspected SGC in a cohort of 91 patients. They found 100% sensitivity of PET/CT for lymph node metastases, compared with 50% for MR imaging.[30] Aside from the determination of simple presence or absence of nodal disease, factors, such as lymph node size, number, and presence

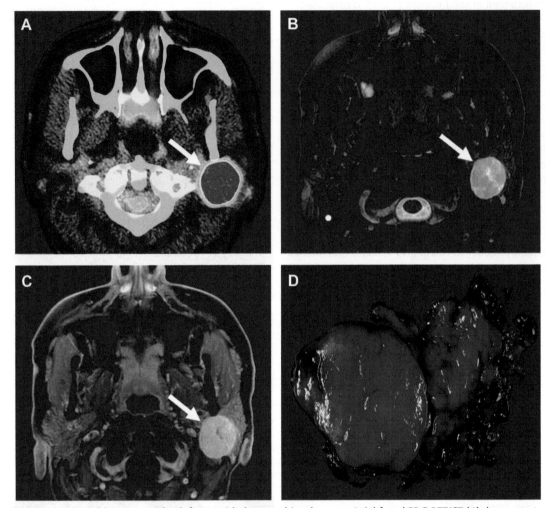

Fig. 4. A 51-year-old woman with a left parotid pleomorphic adenoma. Axial fused FDG PET/CT (*A*) demonstrates a left parotid mass (*arrow*) with intense uptake (SUVmax 11.8). Corresponding axial T2-weighted (*B*) and T1-weighted post-gadolinium (*C*) MR images with fat-suppression demonstrate a circumscribed, rounded mass with heterogeneous T2 hyperintensity and avid enhancement (*arrows*), which was confirmed to be a benign pleomorphic adenoma on surgical resection (*D*).

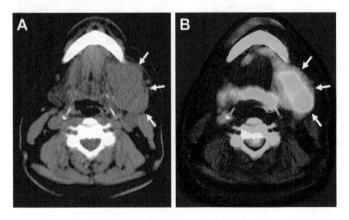

Fig. 5. A 47-year-old man with a left submandibular gland ACC. Axial CT (*A*) and fused FDG PET/CT (*B*) images demonstrate a large left submandibular gland mass (*arrows*) with heterogeneous moderate FDG activity (SUVmax 4.1).

Box 2
TNM staging system for major salivary gland cancers

Tumor (T)

- *pTX:* primary tumor cannot be assessed
- *pT0:* no evidence of primary tumor
- *pTis:* carcinoma in situ
- *pT1:* tumor ≤2 cm without extraparenchymal extension
- *pT2:* tumor greater than >2 cm but ≤4 cm without extraparenchymal extension
- *pT3:* tumor > 4 cm or tumor with extraparenchymal extension
- *pT4a:* tumor of any size invading skin, mandible, ear canal, or facial nerve
- *pT4b:* tumor of any size invading skull base or pterygoid plates or encases carotid artery

Node (N)

- *pNX:* regional lymph nodes cannot be assessed
- *pN0:* no regional lymph node metastasis
- *pN1:* metastasis in a single ipsilateral lymph node ≤3 cm without extranodal extension
- *pN2a:* single ipsilateral lymph node metastasis ≤3 cm with extranodal extension or >3 cm but ≤6 cm without extranodal extension
- *pN2b:* metastasis in multiple ipsilateral lymph nodes ≤6 cm without extranodal extension
- *pN2c:* metastasis in bilateral or contralateral lymph node(s) ≤6 cm without extranodal extension
- *pN3a:* metastasis in a lymph node >6 cm without extranodal extension
- *pN3b:* extranodal extension in a single ipsilateral lymph node >3 cm or single contralateral node or multiple nodes with metastases, any with extranodal extension

Metastasis (M)

- *MX:* indicates distant metastasis cannot be evaluated
- *M0:* indicates the cancer has not spread to other parts of the body
- *M1:* describes cancer that has spread to other parts of the body

Adapted from Amin MB, Edge, S., Greene, F., Byrd, D.R., Brookland, R.K., Washington, M.K., Gershenwald, J.E., Compton, C.C., Hess, K.R., Sullivan, D.C., Jessup, J.M., Brierley, J.D., Gaspar, L.E., Schilsky, R.L., Balch, C.M. AJCC Cancer Staging Manual (8th edition). New York, NY: Springer International Publishing; 2017.

of contralateral disease, also have an impact on N categorization.[31]

PET imaging plays a major role in the identification of distant metastases for the M category (**Fig. 8**), which is simply a binary determination of presence or absence with respect to AJCC staging. In a large single-institution study of patients with major SGC, distant metastases developed in 18.7% of patients, with the lungs the most common site, followed by bone and liver.[32] Distant metastases were more common in men than women. Other predictors of distant metastatic disease included higher T and N categories, high-grade tumor pathology, invasive tumor, and positive tumor margins.

Overall, FDG PET has been shown to be a highly accurate method for both staging[19,33–39] and restaging[33,34,36,37,39] SGC (see **Fig. 7**), with accuracy ranging from 81.8% to 100% in the articles included in a 2015 systematic review.[17] In these studies, PET was shown to change patient management in 15% to 47% of patients with malignant SGTs. In particular, PET has an impact on the surgical approach through identification of locoregional nodal metastases and also alters treatment strategy from primarily surgical to chemoradiation when distant metastases are detected.[17]

Prognostic Value of ^{18}F-fluorodeoxyglucose PET/Computed Tomography

PET/CT provides important prognostic information at baseline assessment for patients with SGC. For example, a retrospective study evaluating 117 patients with salivary carcinoma treated in a multimodal fashion found that the SUVmax of both the primary tumor and locoregional metastatic lymph nodes predicted clinical outcomes. They found an optimal SUVmax cutoff of 7.0; patients with values higher than this in the primary tumor or lymph nodes had less favorable 5-year locoregional control, distant metastasis-free survival (DMFS), progression-free survival (PFS), and overall survival (OS).[40] This same group found that primary tumor SUVmax also is predictive of survival outcomes in SGC patients undergoing definitive intensity-modulated radiation therapy.[41] Suzuki and colleagues[42] noted that higher FDG uptake is associated with lower OS in patients with major SGC in both univariate and multivariate analysis, even after adjusting for pathologic stage.

Other studies have found enhanced prognostication afforded by volumetric metabolic tumor measures, such as metabolic tumor volume (MTV) and total lesion glycolysis (TLG). Ryu and colleagues[43] reviewed 49 patients with

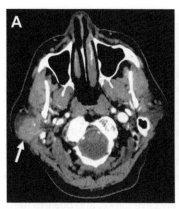
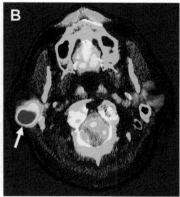
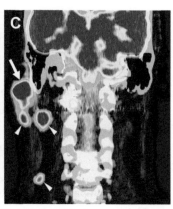

Fig. 6. A 62-year-old man with metastatic right parotid acinic cell carcinoma. Axial contrast-enhanced CT (*A*) demonstrates an enhancing mass within the superficial right parotid gland (*arrow*). Axial (*A*) and coronal (*B*) fused FDG PET/CT images demonstrate marked uptake (SUVmax 10.3) within the parotid mass (*arrows* [*A* and *B*]), and FDG-avid metastatic right cervical lymph nodes (*arrowheads* [*C*]).

intermediate or high-grade SGC treated by definitive surgery with or without adjuvant chemoradiation who underwent PET/CT. In this cohort, higher MTV and TLG were significantly associated with shorter PFS and OS rates, whereas SUVmax was not a significant variable for either PFS or OS.[43] In a study of 75 patients with untreated high-grade SGC, MTV was shown to be an independent predictive factor of metastatic disease on initial staging PET/CT, and, although all PET parameters were significant variables for PFS, only MTV and TLG were significant factors for OS.[44]

Similar conclusions have been reached when looking at specific subsets of SGC, such as ACC. In a retrospective study, including 52 ACC patients with pretreatment FDG PET/CT,

univariate analyses showed that all PET parameters (SUVmax, mean standardized uptake value, peak standardized uptake value, MTV, and TLG) were significantly associated with overall PFS, DMFS, and OS, and, after controlling for clinicopathologic variables, SUVmax remained an independent predictor of PFS, and MTV and TLG were independent predictors of DMFS and disease-specific survival. In this study, patients with MTV greater than 14.8 mL had a 5.9-fold higher risk of distant metastasis and 4.2-fold higher risk of disease specific death than those with lower MTV.[45] Likewise, Gencturk and colleagues[46] studied the prognostic value of quantitative FDG PET/CT parameters in ACC and found that higher SUV ratios (in comparison to blood

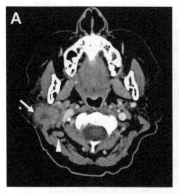
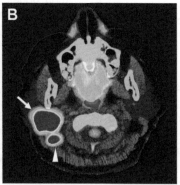
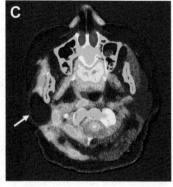

Fig. 7. A 69-year-old woman with a metastatic right parotid squamous cell carcinoma. Axial contrast-enhanced CT (*A*) demonstrates a heterogeneous right parotid mass (*arrow*) and adjacent mildly prominent lymph nodes (*arrowhead*). Axial fused FDG PET/CT (*B*) demonstrates intense uptake (SUVmax 30.6) within the parotid mass (*arrow*) and adjacent lymph nodes (*arrowhead*). The patient underwent total right parotidectomy, select right neck dissection, and abdominal fat graft reconstruction. Follow-up axial fused PET/CT (*C*) showed no residual disease and expected appearance of the fat graft within the parotid bed (*arrow*).

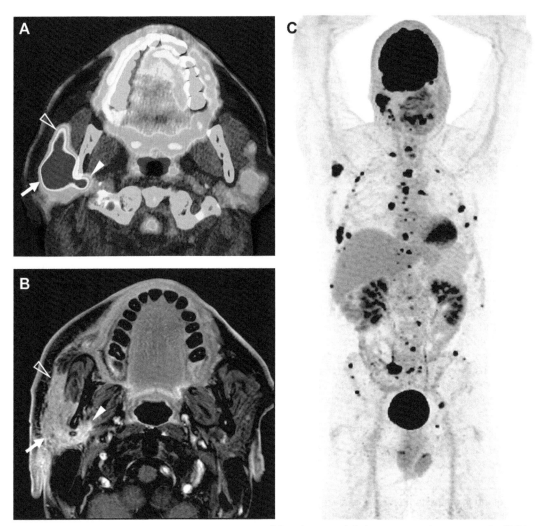

Fig. 8. A 57-year-old man with right parotid ACC. Axial fused PET/CT (*A*) demonstrates intense uptake (SUVmax 12.1) within the parotid mass (*arrow*), with FDG-avid PNS along the right auriculotemporal nerve (*filled arrowhead*) and buccal branch of the right facial nerve (*open arrowhead*). Axial T1-weighted fat-suppressed postcontrast MR imaging (*B*) demonstrates corresponding soft tissue thickening and enhancement in the same regions (*arrow and arrowheads*). FDG PET maximum intensity projection image (*C*) from the same examination as (*A*) demonstrates multiple sites of nodal and osseous metastatic disease.

pool and liver) and MTV and TLG values all predicted DMFS, PFS, and OS independently, whereas SUVmax was an independent predictor of only PFS.

Texture features extracted from PET/CT also have been shown to confer prognostic value. In a study of 85 patients with SGC with high-risk histology, several texture features, including SUV entropy, uniformity, zone-size nonuniformity, and high-intensity zone emphasis, were significantly associated with OS; in this cohort, high SUVmax and high SUV entropy were shown to be the strongest predictors of survival. These factors subsequently were used to create a prognostic model that, when applied to minor SGCs, showed a

significantly higher concordance index for OS than the AJCC stage, WHO risk histology type, or previously published nomograms.[47] Texture analysis of pretreatment FDG PET/CT also has been shown to provide more prognostic information than conventional PET parameters for predicting patient prognosis in locally advanced SGCs treated with interstitial brachytherapy.[48]

^{18}F-fluorodeoxyglucose PET/Computed Tomography in Response Assessment and Surveillance

There has been little published on the role of FDG PET/CT in monitoring response to therapy. In a phase II trial of patients with progressive, locally advanced, and/or metastatic ACC followed by serial PET/CT, PET/CT was useful to demonstrate changes in tumor size and metabolism after treatment.[49] FDG PET/CT also has been shown to be valuable in response assessment in case reports and small series.[50,51]

Studies examining the value of PET/CT for surveillance and assessing local recurrence have arrived at mixed conclusions. For example, in a study including 48 malignant SGT patients undergoing restaging PET/CT, the sensitivity, specificity, and positive and negative predictive values for local recurrence were 83%, 93%, 63%, and 98% for PET versus 67%, 69%, 24%, and 94% for conventional imaging methods, respectively.[33] In contrast, Park and colleagues[36] reviewed 150 PET/CTs performed for surveillance in a cohort of 66 patients with SGTs and found no significant differences in sensitivity, specificity, accuracy, or positive and negative predictive value between PET/CT and conventional imaging for detecting local recurrence, and this has been borne out by other studies as well.[52] As such, there currently is no consensus on the value of PET/CT for surveillance and detecting local recurrence in malignant SGTs compared with conventional imaging.[17]

SPECIAL CONSIDERATIONS
Incidental Parotid Masses on 18F-fluorodeoxyglucose PET/Computed Tomography

Parotid gland incidentalomas have been reported to occur in between 0.3% and 0.45% of PET/CT scans.[25] The reported rate of malignancy in parotid incidentalomas varies widely, from 0% to as high as 50%. In a meta-analysis of focal parotid incidental FDG uptake, the pooled risk of malignancy was 9.6% overall, although the investigators acknowledge that their results may be limited by selection and publication biases.[53] Extra caution should be exercised when seemingly incidental parotid lesions are observed in patients with a history of nonsalivary head and neck malignancy. In a study of 1342 patients with prior head/neck malignancy, the rate of focal parotid uptake was 2.1%, and the malignancy rate of these lesions was 33.3%, composed entirely of metastases.[54] Higher prevalence of focal parotid FDG activity in patients with lung cancer also has been noted in several studies,[55,56] most commonly from Warthin tumors. A significant association between lung cancer and Warthin tumor has been shown in other studies as well,[57] which stands to reason, because smoking is a predisposing factor for both conditions. This also highlights the fact that if focal parotid FDG activity is present on staging PET/CT for lung cancer (see **Fig. 3**), it is more likely to be from a Warthin tumor than metastatic disease.[55]

Perineural Spread

It is important to define the difference between perineural invasion (PNI) and PNS. PNI is a pathologic finding, where there is direct nerve invasion from a contiguous tumor, often involving small nerve branches that are not apparent on imaging studies. Although PNI has a significant negative prognostic value, it is a histologic finding and not something directly visible on PET/CT. In contrast, PNS arises due to PNI but represents the gross radiologic extension along the large nerves in the head and neck.[58] When imaging SGTs with PET/CT, the 2 major cranial nerves that need to be carefully scrutinized are the facial and trigeminal nerves due their extensive innervation of the head and neck and their close proximity to the major and minor salivary glands. Other cranial nerves also can demonstrate PNS in salivary cancers (ie, hypoglossal and oculomotor) but much less frequently.

Given that approximately 40% of PNSs are asymptomatic, imaging plays a vital role in diagnosis.[59,60] In patients with a known parotid malignancy and symptomatic facial weakness, it is critical to locate the facial nerve at the junction of the superficial and deep parotid lobes and then trace proximally to the skull base, where the nerve exits from the stylomastoid foramen. On PET imaging, PNS manifests as linear FDG activity along the expected course of the nerves and their branches, and multiplanar reformatted images can make the detection of PNS easier.[13,61] Careful review of maximum projection images also can increase sensitivity.[62] The stylomastoid foramen should contain the facial nerve surrounded by fat, and, when the fat is missing, this can be an important ancillary sign of PNS on the CT portion of PET/CT. Distally, the facial nerve divides into its 5 major branches within the parotid gland to provide motor function to much of the face (temporal, zygomatic, buccal, marginal mandibular, and cervical).[63] These 5 branches rapidly become too small to clearly follow on CT, MR imaging, or PET studies; so, abnormal PET uptake along their course is highly suspicious for PNS (see **Fig. 8**).

Of the SGT subtypes, ACC and MEC have the greatest predilection for PNS.[62,64] This is particularly true for ACC, in which up to 50% of cases have PNS at the time of diagnosis.[64] The risk of PNS in ACC is higher among lesions that arise from the major salivary glands compared with those from the minor salivary glands.[64] PNS is important to diagnose given its adverse prognostic implications. For example, PNS in MEC has been shown to portend a worse prognosis, independent of histologic grade, tumor size, or positive surgical margins.[65] Likewise, in ACC, PNS is associated with higher rates of local recurrence, distant metastases, and lower 5-year survival.[66] Not only is PNS important to identify for accurate prognostication, but also it has serious implications for treatment planning. Although the primary treatment choice for SGTs is surgery, in cases of parotid tumors, a facial nerve-sparing surgery is possible; thus, it is critical to assess for PNS along cranial nerve VII.[67] Radiation therapy usually is indicated when PNS is present in SGTs because of its association with local recurrence,[68] and PNS often influences the radiation target volume to include coverage of the cranial nerve pathway innervating the primary tumor site.[58]

MR imaging often is the imaging modality of choice for detection of PNS due to superior soft tissue conspicuity compared with CT. Although there have been several case reports and small series indicating that PNS may be depicted on FDG PET,[60,62,69,70] FDG PET and conventional imaging are complementary in evaluation of PNS, with MR imaging the modality of choice for evaluating PNS.[60]

NON–[18]F-FLUORODEOXYGLUCOSE PET RADIOTRACERS

Although the primary use of prostate-specific membrane antigen (PSMA) PET is for evaluation of prostate cancer, PSMA expression has been found in a variety of benign and malignant tumor types, frequently associated with neovasculature in malignant tumors.[71,72] Several case reports have demonstrated ^{68}Ga-PSMA uptake by ACC[73–75]; thus ^{68}Ga-PSMA PET has been explored for evaluation of ACC.[76,77] In 2017, Klein Nulent and colleagues[76] retrospectively examined 9 patients with ACC and found that ^{68}Ga-PSMA was able to detect locally recurrent and metastatic lesions. Three patients underwent both PSMA and FDG PET/CT, and in 1 of these patients, PSMA PET demonstrated local recurrence that was occult on FDG PET/CT. More recently, a prospective phase II study examined the role of PSMA PET/CT in 15 patients with ACC and 10 patients with salivary duct carcinoma, in order to evaluate a potential therapeutic role for ^{177}Lu-PSMA in these patients; 93% of ACC patients and 40% of SDC patients demonstrated PSMA-ligand uptake (defined as tumor/liver ratio >1.0), and PSMA PET detected bone metastases in 2 patients that were occult on CT.[77] This led the investigators to conclude that there may be a role for PSMA radionuclide therapy for second-line treatment in patients with metastatic ACC.

Meirovitz and colleagues[78] recently examined the potential of somatostatin receptor 2 (SSTR2) as a novel therapeutic target in malignant SGTs. Of 63 primary tumors and 14 metastases, they found that all tumors expressed SSTR2 to some extent, including 84% of mucoepidermoid tumors. There was an inverse correlation between SSTR2 and Ki-67 expression. On ^{68}Ga-DOTATATE PET/CT, 40% of patients demonstrated increased radiotracer uptake. This study confirmed SSTR2 expression in SGTs and pointed to a potential role for SSTR2-targeted radiotherapy in some patients with metastatic salivary cancer.[78] Increased ^{68}Ga-DOTA-TOC uptake also has been described in pleomorphic adenoma of the parotid gland.[79]

Head and neck cancers are predominately epithelial in origin and produce cancer-associated fibroblasts, which play a role in aggressive tumor behavior, such as invasion and progression.[80] Cancer-associated fibroblasts overexpress fibroblast activation protein (FAP), which can be imaged by radiolabeled FAP inhibitors, which are labeled most commonly with [68]Ga.[81] Physiologic expression of FAP in healthy tissue is very low, which makes it a potentially ideal agent to image SGTs, given that most other radiotracers, including FDG, have relatively high physiologic salivary gland uptake.[82] FAP PET probes also can be paired with ^{177}Lu and [225]Ac, providing another potential route for delivering targeted radiotherapy to patients with SGTs who may not be candidates for surgery, radiation, or chemotherapy. FAP imaging currently is investigational, but these early results[81] hold promise for broader application to SGTs.

PITFALLS

Many different nonmalignant conditions can cause increased FDG uptake in the salivary glands, including infection, sarcoidosis, and tuberculosis, which can be unilateral or bilateral.[83] Additionally, asymmetric compensatory hypertrophy and increased FDG uptake can be seen with radiation or surgical removal. In the acute period post-radiation, there can be diffusely increased FDG uptake in the radiated area, which can last for up to 3 months.[84] As alluded to previously, many benign tumors of the salivary glands are FDG avid and may be indistinguishable on PET/CT, thus requiring biopsy for definitive diagnosis.[12] Extensive dental amalgam also can cause streak artifact, limiting evaluation in the head and neck, particularly in the submandibular glands.

SUMMARY

PET/CT is useful in the evaluation of SGTs by allowing improved assessment of locoregional and distant metastatic disease compared with conventional imaging and by providing important prognostic information. PET/CT may have utility for detecting local recurrence and assessing therapy response but has not been shown useful in differentiating benign and malignant SGTs. Several non-FDG PET radiotracers demonstrate promise for SGT evaluation and herald a potential theranostic approach to diagnosis and treatment of these tumors.

CLINICS CARE POINTS

- ^{18}F-fluorodeoxyglucose (FDG) PET/computed tomography (CT) is useful for delineating locoregional and distant metastatic disease in malignant salivary gland tumors.

- FDG PET/CT also provides important prognostic information and accurate therapy response assessment in patients with malignant salivary tumors.

- FDG PET/CT has not found to be helpful in differentiating benign and malignant tumors of the salivary glands.

- Focal parotid gland FDG activity in lung cancer patients is more likely to be from Warthin tumor than metastatic disease.

- Perineural spread is most common in adenoid cystic carcinoma and mucoepidermoid carcinoma and presents as linear increased uptake along the expected course of the nerves on FDG PET/CT.

DISCLOSURE

The authors have no relevant financial disclosures or conflicts of interest.

REFERENCES

1.. El-Naggar AK, Chan JKC, Grandis JR, et al. WHO classification of head and neck tumours. Lyon, France: International Agency for Research on Cancer; 2017.

2. Del Signore AG, Megwalu UC. The rising incidence of major salivary gland cancer in the United States. Ear Nose Throat J 2017;96(3):E13–6.

3. Chowdhry AK, McHugh C, Fung C, et al. Second primary head and neck cancer after Hodgkin lymphoma: a population-based study of 44,879 survivors of Hodgkin lymphoma. Cancer 2015; 121(9):1436–45.

4. Saku T, Hayashi Y, Takahara O, et al. Salivary gland tumors among atomic bomb survivors, 1950-1987. Cancer 1997;79(8):1465–75.

5. de Ru JA, Plantinga RF, Majoor MH, et al. Warthin's tumour and smoking. B-ENT 2005;1(2):63–6.

6. Patel DK, Morton RP. Demographics of benign parotid tumours: Warthin's tumour versus other benign salivary tumours. Acta Otolaryngol 2016;136(1):83–6.

7. Noone AM, Cronin KA, Altekruse SF, et al. Cancer incidence and survival trends by subtype using data from the surveillance epidemiology and end results program, 1992-2013. Cancer Epidemiol Biomarkers Prev 2017;26(4):632–41.

8. Britt CJ, Stein AP, Patel PN, et al. Incidental parotid neoplasms: pathology and prevalence. Otolaryngol Head Neck Surg 2015;153(4):566–8.

9. Atula T, Greenman R, Laippala P, et al. Fine-needle aspiration biopsy in the diagnosis of parotid gland lesions: evaluation of 438 biopsies. Diagn Cytopathol 1996;15(3):185–90.

10. Rinaldo A, Shaha AR, Pellitteri PK, et al. Management of malignant sublingual salivary gland tumors. Oral Oncol 2004;40(1):2–5.

11. Carlson ER, Ord RA. Benign pediatric salivary gland lesions. Oral Maxillofac Surg Clin North Am 2016; 28(1):67–81.

12. Friedman ER, Saindane AM. Pitfalls in the staging of cancer of the major salivary gland neoplasms. Neuroimaging Clin N Am 2013;23(1):107–22.

13. Larson CR, Wiggins RH. FDG-PET imaging of salivary gland tumors. Semin Ultrasound CT MR 2019; 40(5):391–9.

14. Thoeny HC. Imaging of salivary gland tumours. Cancer Imaging 2007;7:52–62.

15. Som PM, Curtin HD, Mancuso AA. Imaging-based nodal classification for evaluation of neck metastatic adenopathy. AJR Am J Roentgenol 2000;174(3): 837–44.

16. Alipour R, Smith S, Gupta SK. Utility of metabolic heterogeneity factor in differentiating malignant versus benign parotid uptake on (18)F FDG PET-CT. Am J Nucl Med Mol Imaging 2018;8(6):415–20.

17. Bertagna F, Nicolai P, Maroldi R, et al. Diagnostic role of (18)F-FDG-PET or PET/CT in salivary gland tumors: a systematic review. Rev Esp Med Nucl Imagen Mol 2015;34(5):295–302.

18. Hadiprodjo D, Ryan T, Truong MT, et al. Parotid gland tumors: preliminary data for the value of FDG PET/CT diagnostic parameters. AJR Am J Roentgenol 2012;198(2):W185–90.

19. Kim MJ, Kim JS, Roh JL, et al. Utility of 18F-FDG PET/CT for detecting neck metastasis in patients with salivary gland carcinomas: preoperative planning for necessity and extent of neck dissection. Ann Surg Oncol 2013;20(3):899–905.

20. Ozawa N, Okamura T, Koyama K, et al. Retrospective review: usefulness of a number of imaging modalities including CT, MRI, technetium-99m pertechnetate scintigraphy, gallium-67 scintigraphy and F-18-FDG PET in the differentiation of benign from malignant parotid masses. Radiat Med 2006; 24(1):41–9.

21. Park SB, Choi JY, Lee EJ, et al. Diagnostic Criteria on (18)F-FDG PET/CT for differentiating benign from malignant focal hypermetabolic lesions of parotid gland. Nucl Med Mol Imaging 2012;46(2):95–101.

22. Rubello D, Nanni C, Castellucci P, et al. Does 18F-FDG PET/CT play a role in the differential diagnosis of parotid masses. Panminerva Med 2005;47(3):187–9.

23. Kim BS, Kim SJ, Pak K. Diagnostic value of metabolic heterogeneity as a reliable parameter for differentiating malignant parotid gland tumors. Ann Nucl Med 2016;30(5):346–54.

24. Kendi AT, Magliocca KR, Corey A, et al. Is there a role for PET/CT parameters to characterize benign, malignant, and metastatic parotid tumors? AJR Am J Roentgenol 2016;207(3):635–40.

25. Makis W, Ciarallo A, Gotra A. Clinical significance of parotid gland incidentalomas on (18)F-FDG PET/CT. Clin Imaging 2015;39(4):667–71.

26. Horiuchi C, Tsukuda M, Taguchi T, et al. Correlation between FDG-PET findings and GLUT1 expression in salivary gland pleomorphic adenomas. Ann Nucl Med 2008;22(8):693–8.

27. Ma S, Liu Y. Diagnostic value of fluorine-18 fluorodeoxyglucose positron emission tomography/computed tomography in sublingual and submandibular salivary gland tumors. Mol Clin Oncol 2020; 13(4):27.

28. Toriihara A, Nakamura S, Kubota K, et al. Can dual-time-point 18F-FDG PET/CT differentiate malignant salivary gland tumors from benign tumors? AJR Am J Roentgenol 2013;201(3):639–44.

29. Amin MB, Edge S, Greene F, et al. AJCC cancer staging manual. 8th edition. New York (NY): Springer International Publishing; 2017.

30. Westergaard-Nielsen M, Rohde M, Godballe C, et al. Up-front F18-FDG PET/CT in suspected salivary gland carcinoma. Ann Nucl Med 2019;33(8): 554–63.

31. Abou-Foul AK. Surgical anatomy of the lymphatic drainage of the salivary glands: a systematic review. J Laryngol Otol 2020;1–7.

32. Ali S, Bryant R, Palmer FL, et al. Distant metastases in patients with carcinoma of the major salivary glands. Ann Surg Oncol 2015;22(12):4014–9.

33. Cermik TF, Mavi A, Acikgoz G, et al. FDG PET in detecting primary and recurrent malignant salivary gland tumors. Clin Nucl Med 2007;32(4):286–91.

34. Jeong HS, Chung MK, Son YI, et al. Role of 18F-FDG PET/CT in management of high-grade salivary gland malignancies. J Nucl Med 2007;48(8):1237–44.

35. Kim JY, Lee SW, Kim JS, et al. Diagnostic value of neck node status using 18F-FDG PET for salivary duct carcinoma of the major salivary glands. J Nucl Med 2012;53(6):881–6.

36. Park HL, Yoo Ie R, Lee N, et al. The value of F-18 FDG PET for planning treatment and detecting recurrence in malignant salivary gland tumors: comparison with conventional imaging studies. Nucl Med Mol Imaging 2013;47(4):242–8.

37. Razfar A, Heron DE, Branstetter BFT, et al. Positron emission tomography-computed tomography adds to the management of salivary gland malignancies. Laryngoscope 2010;120(4):734–8.

38. Roh JL, Ryu CH, Choi SH, et al. Clinical utility of 18F-FDG PET for patients with salivary gland malignancies. J Nucl Med 2007;48(2):240–6.

39. Sharma P, Jain TK, Singh H, et al. Utility of (18)F-FDG PET-CT in staging and restaging of patients with malignant salivary gland tumours: a single-institutional experience. Nucl Med Commun 2013; 34(3):211–9.

40. Hsieh CE, Cheng NM, Chou WC, et al. Pretreatment primary tumor and nodal SUVmax values on 18F-FDG PET/CT images predict prognosis in patients with salivary gland carcinoma. Clin Nucl Med 2018;43(12):869–79.

41. Hsieh CE, Ho KC, Hsieh CH, et al. Pretreatment primary tumor SUVmax on 18F-FDG PET/CT images predicts outcomes in patients with salivary gland carcinoma treated with definitive intensity-modulated radiation therapy. Clin Nucl Med 2017; 42(9):655–62.

42. Suzuki H, Tamaki T, Nishio M, et al. Uptake of (18)F-Fluorodeoxyglucose in Major salivary gland cancer predicts survival adjusting for pathological stage. Anticancer Res 2019;39(2):1043–9.

43. Ryu IS, Kim JS, Roh JL, et al. Prognostic value of preoperative metabolic tumor volume and total lesion glycolysis measured by F-18-FDG PET/CT in Salivary Gland Carcinomas. J Nucl Med 2013; 54(7):1032–8.

44. Almuhaimid TM, Lim WS, Roh JL, et al. Pre-treatment metabolic tumor volume predicts tumor metastasis and progression in high-grade salivary gland carcinoma. J Cancer Res Clin Oncol 2018;144(12): 2485–93.

45. Lim WS, Oh JS, Roh JL, et al. Prediction of distant metastasis and survival in adenoid cystic carcinoma using quantitative (18)F-FDG PET/CT measurements. Oral Oncol 2018;77:98–104.

46. Gencturk M, Ozturk K, Koksel Y, et al. Pretreatment quantitative (18)F-FDG PET/CT parameters as a predictor of survival in adenoid cystic carcinoma of the salivary glands. Clin Imaging 2019;53:17–24.

47. Cheng NM, Hsieh CE, Liao CT, et al. Prognostic value of tumor heterogeneity and SUVmax of pretreatment 18F-FDG PET/CT for salivary gland

carcinoma with high-risk histology. Clin Nucl Med 2019;44(5):351–8.

48. Wu WJ, Li ZY, Dong S, et al. Texture analysis of pre-treatment [(18)F]FDG PET/CT for the prognostic prediction of locally advanced salivary gland carcinoma treated with interstitial brachytherapy. EJNMMI Res 2019;9(1):89.

49. Ghosal N, Mais K, Shenjere P, et al. Phase II study of cisplatin and imatinib in advanced salivary adenoid cystic carcinoma. Br J Oral Maxillofac Surg 2011; 49(7):510–5.

50. Holzgreve A, Pfluger T, Schmid I, et al. (18)F-FDG PET/CT for response assessment in pediatric sebaceous carcinoma of the parotid gland. Diagnostics (Basel) 2020;10(11).

51. Correa TS, Matos GDR, Segura M, et al. Second-line treatment of HER2-positive salivary gland tumor: ado-trastuzumab emtansine (T-DM1) after Progression on Trastuzumab. Case Rep Oncol 2018;11(2):252–7.

52. Lee SH, Roh JL, Kim JS, et al. Detection of distant metastasis and prognostic prediction of recurrent salivary gland carcinomas using (18) F-FDG PET/CT. Oral Dis 2018;24(6):940–7.

53. Treglia G, Bertagna F, Sadeghi R, et al. Prevalence and risk of malignancy of focal incidental uptake detected by fluorine-18-fluorodeoxyglucose positron emission tomography in the parotid gland: a meta-analysis. Eur Arch Otorhinolaryngol 2015;272(12): 3617–26.

54. Seo YL, Yoon DY, Baek S, et al. Incidental focal FDG uptake in the parotid glands on PET/CT in patients with head and neck malignancy. Eur Radiol 2015; 25(1):171–7.

55. Barbara RR, Pawaroo D, Beadsmoore C, et al. Parotid incidentalomas on positron emission tomography: what is their clinical significance? Nucl Med Commun 2019;40(3):264–9.

56. Davidson T, Komissar O, Goshen E, et al. Focal fluorine-18 fluorodeoxyglucose-avid parotid findings in patients with lung cancer: prevalence and characteristics. Nucl Med Commun 2016;37(9):969–74.

57. White CK, Williams KA, Rodriguez-Figueroa J, et al. Warthin's tumors and their relationship to lung cancer. Cancer Invest 2015;33(1):1–5.

58. Bakst RL, Glastonbury CM, Parvathaneni U, et al. Perineural invasion and perineural tumor spread in head and neck cancer. Int J Radiat Oncol Biol Phys 2019;103(5):1109–24.

59. Gandhi D, Gujar S, Mukherji SK. Magnetic resonance imaging of perineural spread of head and neck malignancies. Top Magn Reson Imaging 2004;15(2):79–85.

60. Lee H, Lazor JW, Assadsangabi R, et al. An imager's guide to perineural tumor spread in head and neck cancers: radiologic footprints on (18)F-FDG PET, with CT and MRI correlates. J Nucl Med 2019; 60(3):304–11.

61. Chandra P, Purandare N, Shah S, et al. Common patterns of perineural spread in head-neck squamous cell carcinoma identified on fluoro-deoxy-glucose positron emission tomography/computed tomography. Indian J Nucl Med 2016;31(4): 274–9.

62. Paes FM, Singer AD, Checkver AN, et al. Perineural spread in head and neck malignancies: clinical significance and evaluation with 18F-FDG PET/CT. Radiographics 2013;33(6):1717–36.

63. Moonis G, Cunnane MB, Emerick K, et al. Patterns of perineural tumor spread in head and neck cancer. Magn Reson Imaging Clin N Am 2012;20(3):435–46.

64. Barrett AW, Speight PM. Perineural invasion in adenoid cystic carcinoma of the salivary glands: a valid prognostic indicator? Oral Oncol 2009;45(11): 936–40.

65. McHugh CH, Roberts DB, El-Naggar AK, et al. Prognostic factors in mucoepidermoid carcinoma of the salivary glands. Cancer 2012;118(16):3928–36.

66. Vrielinck LJ, Ostyn F, van Damme B, et al. The significance of perineural spread in adenoid cystic carcinoma of the major and minor salivary glands. Int J Oral Maxillofac Surg 1988;17(3):190–3.

67. Bell RB, Dierks EJ, Homer L, et al. Management and outcome of patients with malignant salivary gland tumors. J Oral Maxillofac Surg 2005;63(7):917–28.

68. Garden AS, Weber RS, Morrison WH, et al. The influence of positive margins and nerve invasion in adenoid cystic carcinoma of the head and neck treated with surgery and radiation. Int J Radiat Oncology*Biology*Physics 1995;32(3):619–26.

69. Chandra P, Nath S. Perineural spread of mucoepidermoid carcinoma of parotid gland involving v, vi, and vii cranial nerves demonstrated on positron emission tomography/computed tomography. Indian J Nucl Med 2017;32(3):245–6.

70. Dercle L, Hartl D, Rozenblum-Beddok L, et al. Diagnostic and prognostic value of 18F-FDG PET, CT, and MRI in perineural spread of head and neck malignancies. Eur Radiol 2018;28(4):1761–70.

71. Kinoshita Y, Kuratsukuri K, Landas S, et al. Expression of prostate-specific membrane antigen in normal and malignant human tissues. World J Surg 2006;30(4):628–36.

72. Silver DA, Pellicer I, Fair WR, et al. Prostate-specific membrane antigen expression in normal and malignant human tissues. Clin Cancer Res 1997;3(1): 81–5.

73. de Keizer B, Krijger GC, Ververs FT, et al. 68)Ga-PSMA PET-CT imaging of metastatic adenoid cystic carcinoma. Nucl Med Mol Imaging 2017;51(4): 360–1.

74. Lutje S, Sauerwein W, Lauenstein T, et al. In Vivo Visualization of prostate-specific membrane antigen in adenoid cystic carcinoma of the salivary gland. Clin Nucl Med 2016;41(6):476–7.

75. Uijen MJM, van Boxtel W, van Herpen CML, et al. 68Ga-Prostate-Specific Membrane Antigen-11-Avid Cardiac Metastases in a Patient With Adenoid Cystic Carcinoma, A Rare Presentation of a Rare Cancer. Clin Nucl Med 2020;45(9):716–8.

76. Klein Nulent TJW, van Es RJJ, Krijger GC, et al. Prostate-specific membrane antigen PET imaging and immunohistochemistry in adenoid cystic carcinoma-a preliminary analysis. Eur J Nucl Med Mol Imaging 2017;44(10):1614–21.

77. van Boxtel W, Lutje S, van Engen-van Grunsven ICH, et al. 68Ga-PSMA-HBED-CC PET/CT imaging for adenoid cystic carcinoma and salivary duct carcinoma: a phase 2 imaging study. Theranostics 2020;10(5):2273–83.

78. Meirovitz A, Blum KS, Maly A, et al. The potential of somatostatin receptor 2 as a novel therapeutic target in salivary gland malignant tumors. J Cancer Res Clin Oncol 2021;147(5):1335–40.

79. Laurens ST, Netea-Maier RT, Aarntzen EJHG. 68Ga-DOTA-TOC uptake in pleomorphic adenoma. Clin Nucl Med 2018;43(7):524–5.

80. Wang Z, Tang Y, Tan Y. Cancer-associated fibroblasts in radiotherapy: challenges and new opportunities. Cell Commun Signal 2019;17(1):47.

81. Syed M, Flechsig P, Liermann J, et al. Fibroblast activation protein inhibitor (FAPI) PET for diagnostics and advanced targeted radiotherapy in head and neck cancers. Eur J Nucl Med Mol Imaging 2020; 47(12):2836–45.

82. Luo Y, Pan Q, Yang H, et al. Fibroblast activation protein-targeted PET/CT with (68)Ga-FAPI for imaging IgG4-related disease: comparison to (18)F-FDG PET/CT. J Nucl Med 2021;62(2):266–71.

83. Purohit BS, Ailianou A, Dulguerov N, et al. FDG-PET/CT pitfalls in oncological head and neck imaging. Insights Imaging 2014;5(5):585–602.

84. Kostakoglu L, Hardoff R, Mirtcheva R, et al. PET-CT fusion imaging in differentiating physiologic from pathologic FDG uptake. Radiographics 2004;24(5): 1411–31.

Positron Emission Tomography/Computed Tomography in Thyroid Cancer

Chandrasekhar Bal, MD, DNB, DSc, FAMS, FNASc, FASc[a],*,
Dhritiman Chakraborty, MD, DM[b,1], Dikhra Khan, MD[a]

KEYWORDS

- 18F-FDG PET/CT • Thyroid cancer • Differentiated thyroid cancer • Medullary thyroid cancer
- TENIS

KEY POINTS

- The histologic subtype, receptor status, and tumor biology greatly influence the avidity of fluorine-18-fluorodeoxyglucose-positron emission tomography/computed tomography (18F-FDG PET) in thyroid malignancy.
- 18F-FDG PET/CT has demonstrated value in the assessment of recurrence, radioiodine refractory disease, and prognosis of thyroid malignancy.
- PET/CT using 68Ga-SSA, 68Ga-DOTA-RDG,68Ga-FAPI, and 68Ga-PSMA have a promising role in the management of thyroid cancers.
- 124I PET/CT is a sensitive modality for the detection of recurrent disease, and in dosimetry.

INTRODUCTION

Thyroid cancer represents 2.3% of all new cancer cases in the United States, with an age-adjusted death rate of 0.5 per 100,000 men and women per year based on 2014 to 2018 deaths.[1,2] Thyroid cancer is mainly derived from follicular and parafollicular cells and divided as follows (**Fig. 1**). Despite the advancement in various diagnostic modalities that are used for the early detection and proper treatment of thyroid cancers, some patients have a persistent and recurrent disease with metastatic potential. About 5% to 15% of differentiated thyroid cancer (DTC) and 50% of metastatic DTCs are refractory to RAI treatment contributed by progressive dedifferentiation of DTC and loss of the sodium iodide symporter (NIS) that is required for iodine uptake.[3–5] The role of 18F-FDG and non-FDG PET/CT in different types of thyroid cancer in various stages shall be discussed in this review.

MECHANISM OF 18F-FLUORODEOXYGLUCOSE UPTAKE IN THYROID CANCER

In cancer cells, 18F-FDG being an analog of glucose is transported within the cell through membrane-bound GLUT receptors, particularly GLUT1/2/3, and promptly metabolized to FDG-6-P by hexokinase enzyme. FDG-6-P is trapped in the cell as no further metabolism is possible.

The first 18F-FDG PET scan was performed and published as early as 1987 by Joensuu and Ahonen.[6] In most thyroid tumor cells, GLUT-1 is the major protein mediating the specific transport of 18F-FDG. The expression of GLUT proteins and glucose uptake in thyroid cells is increased with TSH stimulation. TSH-stimulated 18F-FDG uptake is mediated via adenylate cyclase (AC) and cAMP, RAS, PI3K, and AKT. Mitogen-activated protein kinase (MAPK) pathway involving B-type Raf (BRAF), the

[a] Department of Nuclear Medicine, AIIMS, New Delhi 110029, India; [b] Department of Nuclear & Experimental Medical Sciences, Institute of Post Graduate Medical Education and Research/SSKM Hospital, Kolkata, West Bengal, India
[1] Present address: EE-17/5, Sector 2, Salt Lake, Kolkata 700091, India.
* Corresponding author.
E-mail address: drcsbal@gmail.com

PET Clin 17 (2022) 265–283
https://doi.org/10.1016/j.cpet.2021.12.004

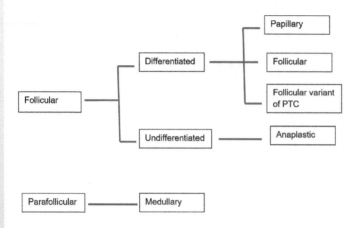

Fig. 1. Types of thyroid cancer.

extracellular signal-regulated kinase, is supposed to steer cell proliferation (**Fig. 2**).

Also, mutation or deletion of onco-suppressor PTEN (phosphatase and tensin homolog) is frequent in thyroid cancers. The lipid phosphatase activity of wild-type PTEN switches off the AKT pathway.[7]

THYROID INCIDENTALOMAS ON FLUORINE-18-FLUORODEOXYGLUCOSE-POSITRON EMISSION TOMOGRAPHY/COMPUTED TOMOGRAPHY

Incidental 18F-FDG uptake, either focal or diffuse, within the thyroid gland has been reported in 1% to 4% of patients undergoing 18F-FDG PET/CT for other reasons.[8,9]

Diffuse incidental FDG uptake commonly represents benign etiology such as thyroiditis.[10–12] Karantanis and colleagues evaluated 4732 patients who underwent FDG PET/CT for other reasons. They found 32 patients with incidental diffuse thyroid uptake and 19/32 patients (59.4%) who were further evaluated had a diagnosis of chronic lymphocytic thyroiditis and FDG uptake attributed to immune lymphocyte infiltration in activated lymphoid tissue (**Fig. 3**).[11]

However, incidental focal FDG uptake shows a 24% to 36% risk of malignancy, most commonly due to papillary thyroid carcinoma (PTC), with pooled malignancy risk was 36.2% (n = 215,-057).[13–15]

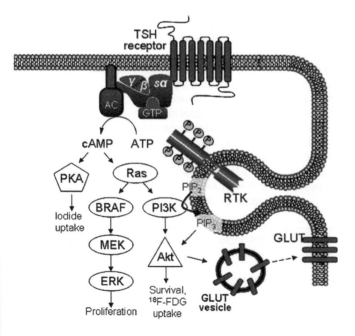

Fig. 2. Mechanism of FDG uptake in thyroid cancer. (*From* Prante O, Maschauer S, Fremont V, Reinfelder J, Stoehr R, Szkudlinski M, Weintraub B, Hartmann A, Kuwert T. Regulation of uptake of 18F-FDG by a follicular human thyroid cancer cell line with mutation-activated K-ras. J Nucl Med. 2009 Aug;50(8):1364-70.).

A   **B**

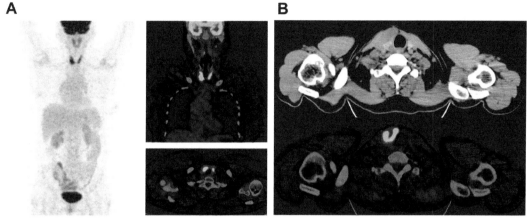

Fig. 3. (*A*): 38-year-old female with invasive ductal carcinoma breast (right) had 18F-FDG PET/CT scan for restaging after 2 years of initial treatment. MIP was normal with diffuse thyroidal FDG uptake. On questioning, she mentioned that she is taking a replacement dose of thyroxin for the last 1 decade for Hashimoto's thyroiditis diagnosed during the first pregnancy. (*B*): This 45-year-old female was investigated for pyrexia of unknown origin with conventional blood work-ups that were normal. The treating unit was advised for 18F-FDG PET/CT scan. The PET scan was normal except for a focal lesion in the right thyroid lobe 3.2 cm × 2 cm with high FDG uptake (SUV-max 22.6). FNAC turned to be classical PTC.

Shie and colleagues showed among the patients with incidental focal thyroid uptake (n = 55,160), 62.1% of patients had the benign disease, 33.2% had cancer, 4.7% were diagnosed as indeterminate nodules, and PTC was the most prevalent (82.2%) histology who had cancer.[16]

Because of this considerable risk, further workup with ultrasound and FNA is necessary. Retrospective review of the impact of 18F-FDG PET detected incidentaloma in the management was conducted by Are and colleagues Thyroid malignancy was noted in 42% (24/57) patients that underwent FNA and 74% (20/27) in those patients who were subjected to operative intervention. The factors that correlated with an increased risk of malignancy were the presence of physical findings and focal or unilateral uptake on PET scans, warranting further investigations followed by the possible operative intervention.[17]

Texture analysis is now a buzzword in imaging science. Solini and colleagues used 18F-FDG-PET/CT texture analysis in 50 patients to predict final diagnosis in thyroid incidentalomas. Among all the textural features tested, skewness showed the best area under the curve (= 0.66). SUV-based parameters resulted in the highest specificity while metabolic tumor volume (MTV), total lesional glycolysis (TLG), skewness, kurtosis, and so forth, showed better sensitivity.[18]

MALIGNANCY RISK PREDICTION OF THYROID NODULES WITH INDETERMINATE CYTOLOGY OR SUSPICIOUS NECK ULTRASONOGRAPHY

About 20% to 30% of patients have indeterminate cytology on FNA, such as the suspicion of a follicular neoplasm. Currently, most of these cases require hemithyroidectomy to exclude malignancy; however, the positive yield (malignancy) is about 25%.[19]

18F-FDG PET/CT could help define the nature of indeterminate thyroid nodules with high sensitivity and NPV; thus, reducing the number of inappropriate thyroidectomies.[20–24] It could play a promising role in the situation of wider unavailability of molecular testing. The existing literature is highly controversial, from very useful to totally useless.[25–27]

Geus-Oei and colleagues studied 18F-FDG-PET/CT in 44 patients with inconclusive FNAC results who later underwent surgery. All 7 patients with DTC had a positive preoperative PET scan, compared with only 13 of 38 patients with benign pathology, indicating an NPV of 100%. These authors proposed that if surgery were conducted only on patients with inconclusive cytology and a positive PET scan, then unnecessary surgery would be reduced by 66%.[25] However, a contrary report was published by Mitchell and colleagues Authors studied 48 patients and reported that only 9 of 15 thyroid carcinomas were FDG-PET positive (sensitivity 60%), while 30 of 33 benign lesions were 18F-FDG-PET/CT negative (specificity 91%), with an NPV of only 83%.[26] Kim and colleagues investigated 46 follicular neoplasms with 18F-FDG-PET/CT and found out all lesions were FDG positive while 21 of 36 operated lesions were benign. These authors concluded that 18F-FDG-PET/CT was of limited value in selecting patients for surgery.[27]

Two meta-analyses by Vrien and colleagues and Wang and colleagues have addressed this issue. The former study reported that the pooled sensitivity, specificity, NPV, and positive predictive value were 95%, 48%, 96%, and 39%, respectively. They found out that in patients with thyroid nodules who had indeterminate FNA biopsy results, a negative 18F-FDG PET scan improved diagnostic accuracy, particularly in patients with lesions greater than 15 mm. The study by Wang and colleagues, which included papers published before 2012, reported a very high pooled sensitivity (about 90%) of 18F-FDG-PET, but lower than that found by Vriens and colleagues and reported that 18F-FDG PET/CT did not add any particular diagnostic benefit to conventional ultrasound. This publication is probably the only study to contradict the findings of many other studies by denying the diagnostic efficacy of 18F-FDG PET/CT in thyroid nodules with undetermined cytology.[28,29]

Rulhman and colleagues studied the usefulness of 18F-FDG PET/CT in the characterization of sonographically suspicious and scintigraphically hypofunctional thyroid nodules; reported its ability to exclude malignancy in the same. The authors retrospectively analyzed 65 patients with cold thyroid nodules on thyroid scan and with suspicious ultrasound features. They noted that 18F-FDG PET/CT had very high sensitivity and NPV in detecting thyroid malignancy (100%) and also showed relatively high specificity and positive predictive values (87% and 61%, respectively).[30]

Thus, it can be summarized that various high-quality studies prove the role of 18F-FDG PET/CT in predicting the risk of malignancy in *thyroid nodules with indeterminate cytology*. However, its role in *thyroid nodules with suspicious ultrasound features* is yet to be established by future studies.

INITIAL DIAGNOSIS IN DIFFERENTIATED THYROID CANCER

ATA 2015 recommends neck ultrasonography as the first-line imaging modality for proper staging of all patients, for malignant or suspicious thyroid nodules, undergoing thyroidectomy. Preoperative use of other imaging modalities, such as contrast-enhanced computed tomography (CECT) and multiparametric magnetic resonance imaging, are only reserved for patients with DTC at high risk of developing distant metastases or those with suspicious mediastinal nodal involvement.[31]

ATA guidelines do not recommend the preoperative use of 18F-FDG PET/CT at all, even when 18F-FDG PET/CT has a high sensitivity (up to 85%) and specificity (up to 95%) for distant metastases in patients with DTC, could be because of only 1% to 4% of patients with DTC initially presents with distant metastasis.[32,33]

Kim and colleagues retrospectively analyzed 60 patients with low or intermediate risk DTC who underwent 18F-FDG PET/CT before thyroidectomy and reported it has very low sensitivity(10%) and NPV(50%) while very high specificity (90%)in detecting lymph node metastases.[34] Two other studies have evaluated the diagnostic accuracy of 18F FDG PET/CT in nodal staging and compared the accuracy of PET with neck ultrasound and contrast-enhanced CT. All 3 modalities had very high specificities, but low sensitivity ($\leq$50%) for lateral LNs, the overall diagnostic accuracy of 18F-FDG PET/CT tended to be higher.[35,36] Neck ultrasound was considered the best methodology for the preoperative assessment of nodal status as it proved to be superior to 18F-FDG PET/CT and contrast-enhanced CT.[37]

Lee and colleagues studied 258 patients with intermediate & high-risk DTC after total thyroidectomy. Authors reported that 18F-FDG PET/CT performed concurrently with 131I therapy detected additional lesions in 14% of patients with DTC. They noted18F-FDG PET/CT is particularly useful after resectioning the recurrent tumor or in patients with stage T3-T4N1 with tumor size greater than 2.0 cm.[38] Another study comprising 90 consecutive patients with either extensive or metastasized high-risk DTC who underwent 18F-FDG PET/CT after the first 131I treatment reported that about 29% of patients had FDG-positive tumor lesions, 36% had RAI-positive lesions, and 8% had matched lesions. 18F-FDG PET/CT refined initial staging in 9% of patients and changed patient management in 21% of cases, mainly in patients with T3bN1 staging and in patients with distant metastases (**Fig. 4**).[39]

The role of 18F-FDG PET/CT in high-risk DTC with aggressive histologic subtypes is not firmly established as only limited experience exists that's to a few case reports or small case series in patients with tall cell,[40] diffuse sclerosing,[41–43] solid/trabecular,[44] and insular variants[45] of DTC.

Thus, it could be noted that preoperatively 18F-FDG PET/CT doesn't have much role in low-risk DTC. In contrast, it may play a significant role in staging (in aggressive histologic subtypes) and probably change the management protocol (in distant metastatic disease).

SUSPICIOUS RECURRENCE IN DIFFERENTIATED THYROID CANCER

Persistently elevated or increasing thyroglobulin (Tg) levels with TSH suppression or TSH

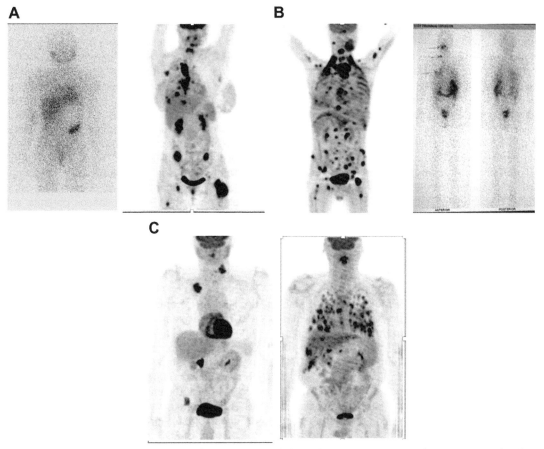

Fig. 4. (*A*): Metastatic PCT in 28-year-old female; posttotal Thyroidectomy 131I-WBS and 18FDG PET/CT (MIP) De novo Radioiodine refractory disease. (*B*): 58-year-old male with extensive metastatic disease. Post-Surgery 131I-WBS & 18FDG PET/CT: Radioiodine Refractory DTC with mixed lesions. (*C*): Follow-up cases of PCT (pT3, N0, M0) who had remnant ablation and undetectable Tg. After 6 to 7 years of recent history of rising Tg and 131I WBS Negative. 18F-FDG PET/CT detected nodal and skeletal metastases in the left panel (first Patient) and pulmonary metastases in right (second patient).

stimulation may represent patients with structural residual or recurrent disease. During follow-up, the rising or persistent abnormal Tg level most often corresponds to loco-regional metastases in the neck. 18F-FDG PET/CT can play a role in the diagnosis of tumor persistence/recurrence. One interesting study by Leboulleux and colleagues evaluated the sensitivity of posttherapeutic 131I WBS versus 18F-FDG PET/CT in patients with elevated serum Tg levels. The authors reported a 16% sensitivity for 131I scan versus 88% for 18F FDG PET/CT. This study included 34 patients with 50% of stage III disease and 24% aggressive histology subtypes. The authors concluded that in patients with the suspicion of recurrence based on Tg levels after a normal postablation WBS, 18F-FDG PET/CT can localize disease than postthera-peutic 131I WBS.[46] A meta-analysis including 789 patients with biochemical residual disease but

negative 131I WBS reported an 18F-FDG PET or PET/CT sensitivity and specificity of 88.5% and 84%, respectively.[47]

Another meta-analysis by Miller and colleagues confirmed that 18F-FDG PET and PET/CT were accurate methods for patients with restaging PTC and reported a pooled sensitivity and speci-ficity of 82% and 84%, respectively.[48] Haslerud and colleagues gathered 17 studies with 905 pa-tients and found the sensitivity and specificity of 18F-FDG PET and PET/CT in restaging DTC to be 80% and 75%, respectively.[49] Diagnostic per-formance of 18F-FDG PET/CT may improve after TSH stimulation,[50] on which the sensitivity of 18F-FDG PET/CT scan only be marginally improved (especially in patients with low Tg values). During the treatment course, a specific sit-uation arises whereby there is no radiologically or clinically evident disease, but Tg levels remain detectable or even significantly elevated (>10 ng/mL), which is called TENIS syndrome (Tg elevated negative iodine scintigraphy).ATA guidelines recommend 18F-FDG PET/CT should be performed when stimulated Tg levels are greater than 10 ng/mL (see Fig. 4).[31]

However, with increasing tumor burden and subsequent rising Tg level, the positivity rate of 18F-FDG PET/CT increases. The true-positive findings have also been reported in 10% to 20% of patients with DTC with Tg levels less than 10 ng/mL.[51,52] An interesting result by Giovanella and colleagues was that a positive 18F-FDG PET/CT scan in patients with biochemical recurrence could be independently predicted by Tg doubling time.[52,53] The accuracy of 18F-FDG PET/CT significantly improved when the Tg doubling time was less than 1 year, irrespective of absolute Tg value.[53]

The clinical utility of Tg monitoring for recurrence can be hampered by the presence of anti-Tg autoantibodies (TgAb) and its interference while Tg measurement. Rising serum TgAb levels during the follow-up of patients with DTC seem to be a good biomarker of persistent or recurrent DTC with undetectable serum Tg levels as TgAb may be produced by the presence of thyroid tissue. A meta-analysis evaluated the diagnostic efficacy of 18F-FDG PET/CT in detecting recurrent and/or metastatic diseases in patients with DTC with progressively and/or persistently elevated TgAb levels and negative 131IWBS and reported pooled sensitivity and specificity to be 84% and 78%, respectively.[54] It is evident from the studies mentioned above that 18F-FDG PET/CT has a role in evaluating DTC relapse.

PROGNOSTIC ROLE IN DIFFERENTIATED THYROID CANCER

An inverse relationship between radioiodine (I-131) and 18F-FDG uptake in thyroid cancer cells is observed during the dedifferentiation process. This phenomenon is called the "flip-flop" phenomenon (Fig. 5), wherein glucose transporters (GLUT1) are upregulated and sodium-iodide symporter (NIS) expression is downregulated.[6] Robbins and colleagues first showed that tumoral phenotype with an intense 18F-FDG uptake is associated with resistance to 131I and, as a result, worsens patient survival. This study retrospectively analyzed the initial 18F-FDG PET/CT uptake in 400 patients with DTC. It assessed the prognostic value of clinical parameters, namely gender, age, serum Tg levels, stage, histology, radioiodine avidity, 18F-FDG-PET positivity, number of FDG-avid lesions, and the glycolytic rate of the most

active lesions. On multivariate analysis, only age and 18F-FDG PET/CT uptake were strongly associated with survival. Also, there were significant inverse relationships between survival and both the glycolytic rate of the most active lesions and the number of FDG-avid lesions.[55] As discussed above, more aggressive and high-grade tumors show a higher FDG uptake than tumors with a favorable prognosis. Also, glucose transporters' expression on the cell membrane is closely related to the grade of malignancy.[56] Thus, 18F-FDG PET/CT has been described as a promising technique in identifying patients with DTC at higher risk of developing distant metastases or patients with distant metastases at higher risk of disease progression.

Nagamachi and colleagues demonstrated the prognostic value of PET/CT in thyroid cancer. The authors noted that, among multiple prognostic factors, only a positive PET/CT uptake (hazard ratio, HR: 5.01, confidence interval (CI): 3.41–6.62) and an age older than 45 years (HR: 4.64, CI: 3.89–5.26) have a significant negative impact on overall survival of patients with DTC on re-staging.[57] Another study by Deandreis and colleagues showed that, compared with radioiodine uptake and histologic or immunohistochemical patterns, 18F-FDG uptake was the only other significant prognostic factor for survival. Even SUV max and the number of FDG avid lesions were also related to prognosis.[58] Negative18F-FDG PET/CT at follow-up predicts a favorable prognosis in patients with DTC with suppressible Tg levels under TSH suppressive therapy < 1 ng/ml.[59] Patients with DTC with a positive follow-up 18F FDG PET/CT scan had shorter overall survival than those who had a negative scan (P < .0001), and in a multivariate Cox regression model, 18F-FDG PET/CT remained associated with overall survival (P < .0001).[60] Considering the special circumstance in patients with DTC and circulating TgAb, the prognostic value of 18F-FDG PET was studied by Bosgrud and colleagues. The authors reported that negative PET results were associated with the absence of active disease and the disappearance of antibodies over time. On the contrary, residual FDG-avid lesions were associated with more aggressive disease and persistently increased TgAb levels.[61]

Patients with DTC with a BRAFV600 E gene mutation have been shown to manifest aggressive behavior. It also carries higher risks of recurrence and disease-specific death. A meta-analysis by Santhanam and colleagues investigated 18F-FDG PET/CT accuracy in detecting residual disease in patients with BRAFV600 E mutated DTC. The presence of this mutation confers a higher

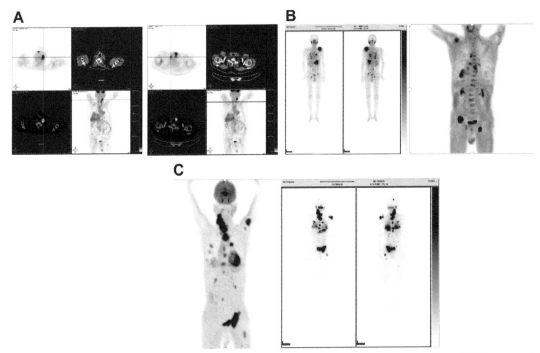

Fig. 5. (*A*): 67-year-old male of PCT on regular follow-up status: post-NTT and postradioiodine ablation. Recently had rising Tg and ^{131}I-negative WBS; Locoregional Recurrence diagnosed by 18F-FDG PET/CT. (*B*): ^{99m}Tc-Pertechnetate Thyroid WBS versus 18FDG PET (MIP). Functioning Well Differentiated Metastatic Follicular Ca Thyroid producing thyrotoxicosis features in this patient. In fact, this patient was referred to us for the radioiodine treatment of hyperthyroidism. 18F-FDG shows uptake in skeletal metastases but missed lung uptake. (*C*): ^{99m}Tc-Pertechnetate Thyroid WBS versus 18FDG PET (MIP). Functioning well-differentiated metastatic follicular Ca thyroid producing thyrotoxicosis features in this patient. In fact, this patient was referred to us for the radioiodine treatment of hyperthyroidism. Interestingly, there was a one-to-one correlation in primary and metastatic sites. It all depends on the degree of differentiation.

likelihood of 18F-FDG avidity compared with its absence.[62]

Identifying Radioiodine Refractory Differentiated Thyroid Cancer and Assessing Its Response to Systemic Therapies

We have already discussed radioiodine refractory thyroid cancer in the previous section. This section will be mainly on the role of 18F-FDG PET/CT in identifying radioiodine refractory DTC and, later on, assessing its response to systemic therapies (**Fig. 6**).18F-FDG PET/CT may detect metastatic disease that is not recognized or only partially seen by posttherapeutic 131I WBS. In these special conditions, treatment by radioiodine should be withheld.[63] Also, 18F-FDG PET/CT may detect newly formed nonradioiodine avid metastases in patients with advanced DTC with unchanged positive posttherapeutic 131I WBS and increasing Tg levels.[64] Furthermore, 18F-FDG PET/CT has been used for the detection of major sites of disease requiring additional localized treatments,

such as surgery, EBRT, radiofrequency ablation, cryotherapy, cement injection, or embolization.

Tyrosine kinase inhibitors (TKI), such as sorafenib and lenvatinib, have been introduced in these RAI refractory progressive patients with DTC. Considering the toxicities of TKI, their use should be reserved for selected metastatic patients.[65] In this scenario, 18F-FDG PET/CT can provide an early assessment of treatment response and seems to be more sensitive in detecting treatment-related changes than other conventional modalities that are based on tumor size (ie, RECIST criteria).[66] Further studies are warranted to assess the ability of 18F-FDG PET/CT to distinguish patients as responders and nonresponders.

Marotta and colleagues evaluated the early metabolic response by using 18F-FDG PET/CT at the baseline and 15 days after treatment initiation and reported a significantly higher baseline average SUVmax who showed disease progression but no correlation with progression-free survival. FDG-PET assessment at the baseline may predict radiological response but not the clinical

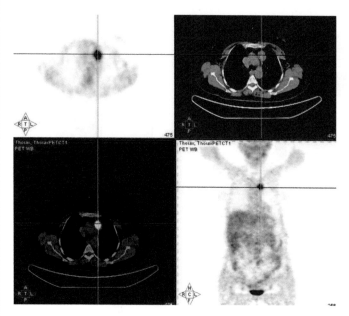

Fig. 6. Known case of PCT in remission following RRA, recently rising serum Tg (from 1.1 raised to 65 ng/mL); Suspected to have loco-regional recurrence. Neck US was negative as well as 131I-WBS. 18F-FDG PET/CT detected a single prevascular node with microcalcification (2.5 cm × 2.1 cm) and SUVmax of 18.5. VATS removed the node and HPE was similar to 1⁰ diagnosis. Six-weeks later Tg become undetectable.

outcome.[67] Carr and colleagues conducted a phase II trial to evaluate the efficacy of sunitinib in patients with metastatic RAI-refractory thyroid cancer. The authors assessed the early response with 18F-FDG-PET/CT after 7 days of treatment. They observed a high disease response rate (78%) and a significant association between an average SUV percent change and the RECIST response criteria. Patients with some response (partial/complete response and stable disease) showed a significantly greater decline in SUVs values than patients with progressive disease. Decrease SUV means that an early 18F-FDG-PET/CT in patients on TKI treatment could be an early indicator of response and may identify patients unlikely to respond to Sunitinib.[68]

Ahmaddy and colleagues assessed the role of 18F-FDG PET/CT in the monitoring of functional tumor response compared with the morphologic response in advanced radioiodine refractory differentiated thyroid carcinoma treated with Lenvatinib. The authors reported that tumor response assessment by 18F-FDG PET outperforms morphologic response assessment by CT in patients with advanced radioiodine refractory DTC treated with Lenvatinib, which seems to be correlated with clinical outcomes.[69]

More studies are needed to validate the role of 18F-FDG PET/CT in identifying radioiodine-refractory disease to exclude metastatic patients from RAI administration. The routine usage of 18F-FDG PET/CT in predicting the efficacy of TKI is not strongly supported by currently published studies, as the present literature has conflicting results. Therefore, more prospective investigations are necessary to shed light on this indication.

68GA-DOTA-SSTR ANALOG POSITRON EMISSION TOMOGRAPHY/COMPUTED TOMOGRAPHY

DTC cells have a high expression of Sstr2, Sstr3, and Sstr5.[70,71] Three studies have compared the diagnostic performance of 68Ga-labeled SSTR analogs (DOTATOC, DOTANOC, DOTALAN PET/CT) with 18F-FDG PET/CT staging iodine-negative DTC so far.[72–74] SSTR-targeted 68Ga-DOTATATE PET/CT imaging may be considered to explore the possibility of PRRT; if the metastatic lesions show high-grade uptake.[75] Considering that a relatively low fraction of non–avid iodine patients with DTC have high expression of SSTRs, comprehensive patient selection using 68Ga-DOTA-SSTR PET/CT seems inevitable, in this situation, it can be used as a reliable tool for staging and therapy assessment (**Fig. 7**).[75]

68GA-DOTA-RGD2 POSITRON EMISSION TOMOGRAPHY/COMPUTED TOMOGRAPHY IN RADIOIODINE REFRACTORY DIFFERENTIATED THYROID CANCER

Role of 68Ga-DOTA-(RGD)2 PET/CT directed toward integrin αvβ3, neoangiogenesis biomarker was explored by Parihar and colleagues Authors compared the diagnostic accuracy of 18F-FDG PET/CT and 68Ga-DOTA-(RGD)2 PET/CT in RAIR-DTC.[76] 18F-FDG PET/CT detected a total of 123 lesions, with an overall sensitivity, specificity, and accuracy of 82.3%, 100%, and 86.4%,

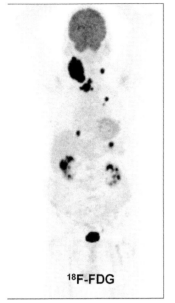
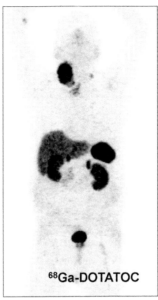

18F-FDG

68Ga-DOTATOC

Fig. 7. Head-to-head comparison of ^{68}Ga-DOTA-TOC and ^{18}F-FDG PET (MIP). 18F-FDG detected more lesions than former tracer. However, for later theranostic applications are potential benefits.

respectively. 68Ga-DOTA-(RGD)2 PET/CT showed similar sensitivity with higher specificity and overall accuracy than 18F-FDG PET/CT in detecting lesions in patients with RAIR-DTC. As most patients (82.1%) were positive on the 68Ga-DOTA-(RGD)2 PET/CT scan, a novel 177Lu-based theranostics can potentially treat these patients.

REAL-TIME USG-FLUORINE-18-FLUORODEOXYGLUCOSE-POSITRON EMISSION TOMOGRAPHY/COMPUTED TOMOGRAPHY FUSION IMAGING

Ultrasonography is an important tool in the initial evaluation of thyroid nodules and subsequently in the follow of DTC. Ballal and colleagues[77] evaluated the role of real-time ultrasonography fused with 18F-FDG PET/CT for intervention. Volume Navigation is a new software option that provides advanced clinical tools possible by facilitating real-time fusion of USG with PET/CT, MRI, and CT examinations for additional information and patient management. All patients underwent 18F-FDG PET/CT and fusion USG-PET/CT within a 1-week interval. The fusion process provides complete information regarding the true loco-regional positive disease burden lesion by lesion and distant metastatic status, which will aid in the precise management of these patients (**Fig. 8**).

124I-PET PET/CT

Dosimetry-based RAIin thyroid cancer is always fraught with controversy. However, the availability

and transportability of 124I, with a physical half-life of 4.2 days, allows repeated acquisitions over days to evaluate the residence time required to quantify the radioactivity in the tumors and normal organs. This unique feature of 124I specifically makes124I-PET the best tool for dosimetry studies described by Freudenberg.[78] A study by Van Nostrand and colleagues showed the superiority of 124I-PET compared with diagnostic planar 131I WBS.[79] In multiple other studies, there have been discrepancies between 131I WBS and 124I-PET.[80–84] Further exploration into this area is needed to use 124I PET for clinical purposes routinely.

FLUORODEOXYGLUCOSE-POSITRON EMISSION TOMOGRAPHY/COMPUTED TOMOGRAPHY IN HÜRTHLE CELL THYROID CARCINOMA

Hürthle cell thyroid carcinoma (HCTC) is defined as when Hürthle cells constitute more than 50% of cells, and pure Hürthle cell is about 100% cells are Hürthle cells. As Hürthle cells do not concentrate iodine, pure Hürthle cell carcinoma is noniodine avid. Thus, it behaves aggressively with a high risk of metastasis and a worse prognosis when compared with DTC.[85] The mainstay of therapy is surgery, which may or may not be accompanied by external beam radiotherapy (EBRT). Pryma and colleagues studied 44 patients with HCTC, out of which 24 were positive and 20 were negative on FDG-PET scans giving a sensitivity and a specificity of about 95%.[86]

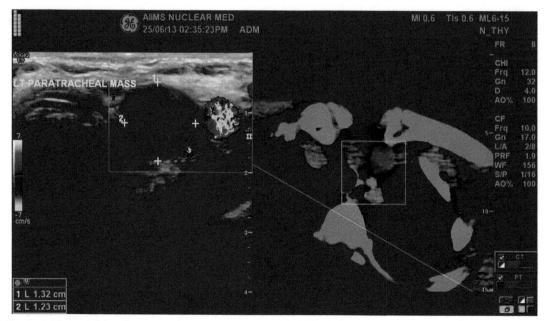

Fig. 8. A 33-year-old male, PTC underwent total thyroidectomy and nodal dissection. Follow-up radioiodine scan was negative for disease, but, the serum Tg level was elevated (16.9 ng/mL). Sonogram to the left and corresponding coregistered 18F-FDG PET/CT image to the right show a left paratracheal lymph node with suspicious features on neck sonography and avid uptake of FDG on PET/CT. USG-FNAC of the lymph node showed features consistent with PTC. This image demonstrates an example of true positive USG and 18F-FDG PET/CT images.

FLUORINE-18-FLUORODEOXYGLUCOSE-POSITRON EMISSION TOMOGRAPHY/COMPUTED TOMOGRAPHY IN POORLY DIFFERENTIATED THYROID CANCER

Poorly differentiated thyroid cancer (PDTC) is a histologic subtype between DTC and anaplastic thyroid cancer (ATC). PDTC preserves some markers of differentiation, such as Tg and thyroid transcription factor1 (TTF1), and at the same time shows some microscopic features of anaplasia.[87] Usually, PDTC is FDG positive tumor with an intermediate GLUT1 expression with uptake between ATC and DTC because of the "flip-flop" phenomenon.[88,89] Thyrotropin increases FDG uptake in PDTC cells; therefore, performing 18F-FDG PET/CT scan under TSH stimulation may be more efficient.[90] Radioiodine therapy may not be useful because of poor tracer uptake in PDTC; rather, surgery and EBRT could be considered.

No particular study analyzed the role of FDG-PET in PDCT only (**Fig. 9**). Some authors suggested using 18F-FDG PET or PET/CT in staging patients with PDTC, specifically in postthyroidectomy staging of high-risk patients.[51]

FLUORINE-18-FLUORODEOXYGLUCOSE-POSITRON EMISSION TOMOGRAPHY/COMPUTED TOMOGRAPHY IN ANAPLASTIC THYROID CANCER

ATC accounting for less than 5% of all thyroid carcinomas, often diagnosed in older patients and usually has a rapid onset of growth. The unique feature of ATC is an extensive local invasion with a median survival time is about 6 to 8 months.[91,92] It is an aggressive thyroid tumor arising from follicular cells that have lost the ability to take up iodine and Tg production. It shows high glucose metabolism and, thus, high FDG uptake.[88,89]

18F-FDG PET/CT in ATC was used for resectability evaluation and follow-up, with a higher sensitivity than CT alone (**Fig. 10**). ATA recommends 18F-FDG PET/CT in assessing metastatic patients, especially bone lesions, and recommends therapy response assessment after 3 to 6 months in patients with no disease or persistent structural disease as a guide to a further course of action.[93]

Poisson and colleagues conducted a study on 20 patients with ATC with 18F-FDG PET/CT for initial staging and follow-up. SUVmax and

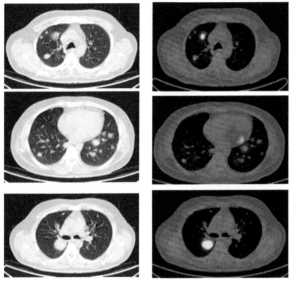

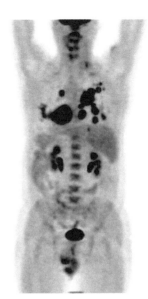

Fig. 9. 45-year-old male had an Rt STN for 20 yrs, Developed cervical nodal mets, FNAC: PCT. CXR-NAD and CECT chest- normal; NTT with nodal clearance in July 2005; HPE: primary tumor PCT with one of the node showing squamous metaplasia. 100 mCi ^{131}I administered in October, PT scan: residual only, no lung uptake. Six months later in Dec CXR & CECT shows cannon balls in lungs, Tg repeated several times: UD. Feb 2006: Posttherapy ^{18}F-FDG PET/CT Progressive Disease in Chest.

functional volume were predictive factors for survival in univariate analysis. Conversely, in bivariate analysis, only functional volume is a prognostic factor. After treatment, a negative 18F-FDG PET/CT scan confirmed complete long-term remission. The authors suggested using 18F-FDG PET/CT in ATC during initial staging, early and long-term follow-up, and assessing treatment response.[94]

Bogsrud and colleagues studied the role of 18F-FDG PET/CT in the management of patients with ATC. They compared it with other diagnostic modalities (CT, ultrasound, magnetic resonance imaging, bone scan, and histology) and clinical follow-up. In all 16 patients included, 18F-FDG PET/CT was positive for primary tumors and influenced the clinical management in 50% of patients. These authors suggested that 18F-FDG PET/CT could improve disease staging and change clinical management of patients with ATC.[95]

To summarize, 18F-FDG PET/CT should be used in patients with ATC in initial staging and in the follow-up after surgery to evaluate metastatic disease in addition to conventional imaging.

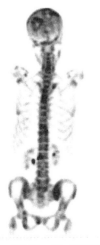

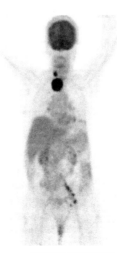

Fig. 10. 69-year-old man had a recent history of thyroid nodule (right lobe) which was rapidly growing (7.5 cm × 8.2 cm), hard on palpation, and fixed to the underlying structure. FNA revealed spindle cell anaplastic thyroid carcinoma. The treating surgeon advised for 18F-FDG PET/CT scan to rule out distant metastases. Interestingly, 18F-FDG revealed primary tumor with ipsilateral node but missed skeletal metastases that were picked-up in 18F- sodium fluoride PET/CT scan. Patient was referred to medical oncologist for palliative care.

18F Fluoride PET/CT   18F FDG PET/CT

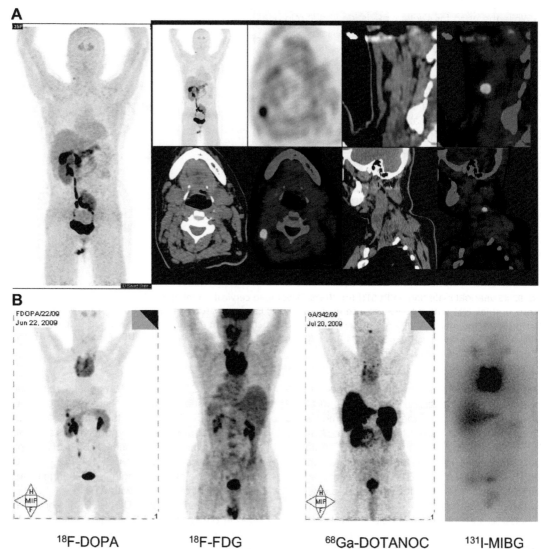

^{18}F-DOPA ^{18}F-FDG ^{68}Ga-DOTANOC ^{131}I-MIBG

Fig. 11. (A): 36-year-old female with sporadic MTC diagnosed 5 years back. She had total thyroidectomy and bilateral neck dissection. Her serum Calcitonin was less than 5 pg/mL all these years. Recently her serum Calcitonin raised to 130 pg/mL. Her 18FDG and 68Ga-DOTANOC PET/CT were negative. However, her 18FDOPA PET/CT detected right cervical level V node 8 mm largest diameter. After the selective excision of the node, the serum calcitonin become less than 5 pg/mL and HPE: confirmed metastatic MTC. (B): Various radiotracers to diagnose and treat recurrent MTC in mediastinum.

POSITRON EMISSION TOMOGRAPHY/ COMPUTED TOMOGRAPHY IN MEDULLARY THYROID CANCER

Medullary thyroid cancer (MTC) is a neuroendocrine tumor, comprises 1% to 2% of thyroid malignancies. MTC originates from the neural crest-derived parafollicular C cells of the thyroid gland.[96] The majority of MTC presents as sporadic and 25% to 30% as hereditary form as part of multiple endocrine neoplasia 2 (MEN2) syndromes. The

mainstay of treatment is surgery, total thyroidectomy, and risk-adapted neck dissections.[97] The role of functional radionuclide imaging in PET/CT is limited in the preoperative setting. During postoperative increase in serum levels of MTC markers with corresponding negative or inconclusive morphologic imaging, PET/CT is used to detect and localize the recurrent disease.

Patient-based detection rate of 18F-FDG PET or PET/CT in recurrent MTC ranges from 59% to 69%.[98,99] 18F-FDG PET/CT shows improved

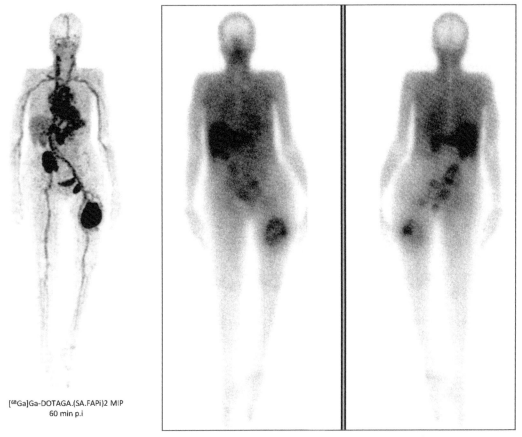

[68Ga]Ga-DOTAGA.(SA.FAPi)2 MIP
60 min p.i

Fig. 12. 45-year-old female presented in 2002 with neck swelling for 12 to 13 years. H/o Right NOF # in Nov 2001 & Left femur shaft #. NTT in 2002; HPE: Follicular Ca thyroid. 131I WBS (2002) Remnant and functioning mets. PT scan – Extensive skeletal metastasis 2002 to 2007 : 1.4 Ci given; Tg was less than 10 till 2016. EBRT to left femur mets. She achieved a good partial response. In 2019, her Tg becomes greater than 30,000 ng/mL. 18F-FDG PET/CT: Lung and skeletal metastasis. TKI- Lenvatinib 24 mg PO started; patient could not tolerate Lenvatinib even after dose reduction to 10 mg OD. 68Ga-DOTAGA-(SA.FAPI)2 PET/CT showed excellent skeletal uptake. On humanitarian ground, we got ethical clearance to try theranostics using 177Lu-DOTAGA-(SA.FAPI)2. 177Lu-FAPi DIMER POST THERAPY SCANS at 72-hours postinjected activity 41 mCi.

sensitivity improved if the patient has shorter serum calcitonin and CEA doubling times.[100,101]

L-type amino acid transporter (LAT) expression and AADC activity are upregulated in MTC; this fact is exploited in 18F-FDOPA PET/CT imaging and expected to help diagnose metastatic sites.18F-FDOPA uptake mostly depends on calcitonin levels, and its sensitivity varies from 47% up to 83%.[100] Slavikova and colleagues showed 18F-FDOPA accuracy becomes significant if calcitonin is greater than 150 pg/mL.[102] Treglia and colleagues reported 100% sensitivity of 18F-DOPA PET/CT for nodal lymph disease.[103] Another added advantage of 18F-FDOPA PET/CT is detecting a synchronous pheochromocytoma in patients with MEN2 (**Fig. 11**).

NET cells in MTC may overexpress somatostatin receptors (SSTRs). 68Ga-SSA PET/CT confirms the SSTR expression, assesses disease burden, and a necessary prerequisite PRRT using therapeutic radionuclides like 177Lu, 90Y, 225Ac in recurrent/metastatic MTC. The detection rate of 68Ga-SSA PET or PET/CT is 63.5% in suspected recurrent MTC and improves with an increasing calcitonin level.[104] Furthermore, for response assessment after PRRT, it can be used as a tool.[105]

In summary, 18F-FDOPA PET/CT is preferred as a first-line procedure in the evaluation of MTC. In case of negative or unfeasible 18F-FDOPA PET/CT, 18F-FDG PET/CT should be performed, particularly if calcitonin and CEA levels are rapidly rising (ie, doubling time < 1 year) or aggressive behavior of the disease is expected (eg, CEA levels disproportionately high compared with calcitonin levels). 68Ga-SSA PET/CT could be considered in selected cases with inconclusive anatomic imaging, 18F-FDOPA, and 18F-FDG PET/CT results and assess the feasibility of PRRT.

POSITRON EMISSION TOMOGRAPHY/COMPUTED TOMOGRAPHY IN THYROID LYMPHOMA

Primary thyroid lymphoma (PTL) accounts for 1% to 5% of all thyroid malignancies and 1% to 2.5% of all lymphomas.[106] The usual treatment is chemotherapy with or without radiotherapy. Surgery has little role in managing PTL, limited to making tissue diagnosis, or very rarely in patients with severe airway obstruction. 18F-FDG PET/CT showed higher SUVmax and lowered CT density than chronic lymphocytic thyroiditis.[107] Like lymphoma in all other organs, 18F-FDG PET/CT is used in primary staging, assessing response, and detecting recurrence in PTL.

NONSTANDARD POSITRON EMISSION TOMOGRAPHY/COMPUTED TOMOGRAPHY IN THYROID MALIGNANCY

68Ga-PSMA PET/CT was explored in PDTC and ATC with the intent of theranostic application using 177Lu, 90Y, and 225Ac labeled radiopharmaceuticals.[108,109] One study demonstrated the feasibility of anti-CEA immune-PET using a 68Ga-labelled radiotracer (IMP288) in patients with MTC.[110] Another study evaluated the possible role of PET using the amino acid tracer 11C-methionine in patients with recurrent MTC.[111] Localization of recurrent or metastatic lesions in patients with DTC with TENIS was tried with 68Ga- fibroblast activation protein inhibitor (FAPI) PET/CT (**Fig. 12**) with theranostic potential.[112] However, none of these proved to have an established role.

During the time of interpretations of different PET/CT scans, pitfalls should be taken care of adequately (**Box 1**).

SUMMARY

18F-FDG PET/CT is the most important PET radiotracer for diagnosing recurrences of DTC to identify radioiodine refractory disease. Its use has also been studied in aggressive variants such as tall cell, diffuse sclerosing, solid/trabecular, and an insular variant of DTC. 18F-FDOPA has been proved to be more sensitive, specifically in diagnosing metastases when CT >150 pg/mL, compared with 18F-FDG. 68Ga-DOTATOC PET/CT has the potential to identify patients for PRRT in case of significant lesion uptake in the medullary thyroid cancer and 60% cases of radioiodine refractory DTC. Currently, 124I PET is being used for dosimetry, but its potential use as therapeutic applications needs further investigations. Interestingly, other newer PET radiotracers, particularly FAPI or DOTA-RGD dimer-based theranostics that involve different metabolic pathways or receptor statuses, are being studied.

Some unmet needs of 18F-FDG PET/CT in thyroid carcinoma deserve more attention in the future.

a. Should an ^{18}FDG PET scan be used for 1^0Dx of STN whereby FNAC has Follicular Neoplasm?
b. Are all hot nodules on ^{18}FDG PET scan Thy malignancy?
c. Should all patients with DTC undergo an ^{18}FDG PET scan for prognostications? Patients who are both iodine WBS-negative and ^{18}FDG PET-negative seem to have a good prognosis.

Box 1
Pitfalls of 18F-FDG PET/CT

18F-FDG uptake due to benign causes:

- Symmetric and diffuse
  - Diffuse goiter or multinodular goiter
  - Autoimmune thyroid disorder
  - Hashimoto thyroiditis
  - Graves disease
  - Hypothyroidism with or without levothyroxine replacement
- Focal
  - Nonspecific
  - Benign thyroid nodule

Focal FDG uptake may be misinterpreted as metastatic lymphadenopathy (neck USG/CT correlation required). Considering the malignant potential metabolically active nodule with low-risk TIRAD features further work up is required.

Increased diffuse FDG uptake in colon in patients with Sorafenib

Pitfalls of 68Ga-PSMA PET/CT

Diffuse: Hypothyroidism

Focal: Incidentaloma

Pitfalls of 68Ga-SSA PET/CT

- Symmetric and diffuse
  - Physiologic
  - Diffuse goiter or multinodular goiter
  - Autoimmune thyroid disorder
  - Hashimoto thyroiditis
  - Hypothyroidism

CLINICS CARE POINTS

- TENIS and Radioiodine refractory DTC are not same.
- Dediffferentiated DTC may not produce sufficient thyroglobulin to be called TENIS.
- 18FDG PET/CT should be used judiciously because of significant risk of false positive PET Scan leading to host of unnecessary medical expenses and patient anxiety.

DISCLOSURE

The authors have nothing to disclose.

REFERENCES

1. Reiners C, Geling M, Luster M, et al. Epidemiologie des Schilddrüsenkarzinoms. Onkologe (Berl) 2005; 11:11–9.
2. Howlader N, Noone AM, Krapcho M, et al (eds). SEER Cancer Statistics Review, 1975-2018. Available at: https://seer.cancer.gov/statfacts/html/thyro.html. Accessed May 10. 2021.
3. Zarnegar R, Brunaud L, Kanauchi H, et al. Increasing the effectiveness of radioactive iodine therapy in the treatment of thyroid cancer using Trichostatin A, a histone deacetylase inhibitor. Surgery 2002;132:984–90.
4. Worden F. Treatment strategies for radioactive iodine-refractory differentiated thyroid cancer. Ther Adv Med Oncol 2014;6:267–79.
5. Xing M, Haugen BR, Schlumberger M. Progress in molecular-based management of differentiated thyroid cancer. Lancet 2013;381:1058–69.
6. Joensuu H, Ahonen A. Imaging of metastases of thyroid carcinoma with fluorine-18 fluorodeoxyglucose. J Nucl Med 1987;28:910–4.
7. Prante O, Maschauer S, Fremont V, et al. Regulation of uptake of 18F-FDG by a human follicular thyroid cancer cell line with mutation-activated K-ras. J Nucl Med 2009;50(8):1364–70.
8. Pagano L, Samá MT, Morani F, et al. Thyroid incidentaloma identified by 18F-fluorodeoxyglucose positron emission tomography with CT (FDG-PET/CT): clinical and pathological relevance. Clin Endocrinol (Oxf) 2011;75:528–34.
9. Nishimori H, Tabah R, Hickeson M, et al. Incidental thyroid "PETomas": clinical significance and novel description of the self-resolving variant of focal FDG-PET thyroid uptake. Can J Surg 2011;54:83–8.
10. Kurata S, Ishibashi M, Hiromatsu Y, et al. Diffuse and diffuse-plus-focal uptake in the thyroid gland identified using FDG-PET: prevalence of thyroid cancer and Hashimoto's thyroiditis. Ann Nucl Med 2007;21:325–30.
11. Karantanis D, Bogsrud TV, Wiseman GA, et al. Clinical significance of diffusely increased 18F-FDG uptake in the thyroid gland. J Nucl Med 2007;48: 896–901.
12. Chen W, Parsons M, Torigian DA, et al. Evaluation of thyroid FDG uptake incidentally identified on FDG-PET/CT imaging. Nucl Med Commun 2009; 30:240–4.
13. Treglia G, Bertagna F, Sadeghi R, et al. Focal thyroid incidental uptake detected by 18F-fluorodeoxyglucose positron emission tomography: a meta-analysis on prevalence and malignancy risk. Nuklearmedizin 2013;52:130–6.
14. Kim H, Kim SJ, Kim IJ, et al. Thyroid incidentalomas on FDG PET/CT in patients with non-thyroid cancer: a large retrospective monocentric study. Onkologie 2013;36:260–4.
15. Bertagna F, Treglia G, Piccardo A, et al. F18-FDG-PET/CT thyroid incidentalomas: a wide retrospective analysis in three Italian centers on the significance of focal uptake and SUV value. Endocrine 2013;43:678–85.
16. Shie P, Cardarelli R, Sprawls K, et al. Systematic review: prevalence of malignant incidental thyroid nodules identified on fluorine-18 fluorodeoxyglucose positron emission tomography. Nucl Med Commun 2009;30(9):742–8.
17. Are C, Hsu JF, Schoder H, et al. FDG-PET detected thyroid incidentalomas: Need for further investigation. Ann Surg Oncol 2007;14:239–47.
18. Sollini M, Cozzi L, Pepe G, et al. [18F]FDG-PET/CT texture analysis in thyroid incidentalomas: preliminary results. Eur J Hybrid Imaging 2017;1(1):3.
19. Keutgen XM, Filicori F, Fahey TJ 3rd. Molecular diagnosis for indeterminate thyroid nodules on fine-needle aspiration: advances and limitations. Expert Rev Moldiagn 2013;13(6):613–23.
20. Kresnik E, Gallowitsch HJ, Mikosch P, et al. Fluorine-18-fluorodeoxyglucose positron emission tomography in the preoperative assessment of thyroid nodules in an endemic goiter area. Surgery 2003;133(3):294–9.
21. Sebastianes FM, Cerci JJ, Zanoni PH, et al. Role of 18F fluorodeoxyglucose positron emission tomography in preoperative assessment of cytologically indeterminate thyroid nodules. J Clinendocrinolmetab 2007;92:4485–8.
22. Hales NW, Krempl GA, Medina JE. Is there a role for fluorodeoxyglucose positron emission tomography/computed tomography in cytologically indeterminate thyroid nodules? Am J Otolaryngol 2008;29:113–8.
23. Traugott AL, Dehdashti F, Trinkaus K, et al. Exclusion of malignancy in thyroid nodules with indeterminate fine-needle aspiration cytology after

negative 18Ffluorodeoxyglucose positron emission tomography: an interim analysis. World J Surg 2010;34:1247–53.

24. Giovanella L, Suriano S, Maffioli M, et al. 18FDG-positron emission tomography/computed tomography (PET/CT) scanning in thyroid nodules nondiagnostic cytology. Clin Endocrinol 2011;74:644–8.

25. de Geus-Oei LF, Pieters GF, Bonenkamp JJ, et al. 18F-FDG PET reduces unnecessary hemithyroidectomies for thyroid nodules with inconclusive cytologic results. J Nucl Med 2006;47(5):770–5.

26. Mitchell JC, Grant F, Evenson AR, et al. Preoperative evaluation of thyroid nodules with 18FDG-PET/CT. Surgery 2005;138(6):1166–74.

27. Kim JM, Ryu JS, Kim TY, et al. 18F-fluorodeoxyglucose, positron emission tomography does not predict malignancy in thyroid nodules cytologically diagnosed follicular neoplasm. J Clin Endocrinol Metab 2007;92:1630–4.

28. Wang N, Zhai H, Lu Y. Is fluorine-18 fluorodeoxyglucose positron emission tomography useful for the thyroid nodules with indeterminate fine-needle aspiration biopsy? A meta-analysis of the literature. J Otolaryngol Head Neck Surg 2013;42(1):38.

29. Vriens D, de Wilt JH, van der Wilt GJ, et al. The role of [18F]-2-fluoro-2-deoxy-d-glucose-positron emission tomography in thyroid nodules with indeterminate fine-needle aspiration biopsy: systematic review and meta-analysis of the literature. Cancer 2011;117(20):4582–94.

30. Ruhlmann M, Ruhlmann J, Görges R, et al. 18F-Fluorodeoxyglucose positron emission tomography/computed tomography may exclude malignancy in sonographically suspicious and ScintigraphicallyHypofunctional thyroid nodules and reduce unnecessary thyroid Surgeries. Thyroid 2017;27(10):1300–6.

31. Haugen BR, Alexander EK, Bible KC, et al. 2015 American Thyroid Association management guidelines for adult patients with thyroid nodules and differentiated thyroid cancer: the American Thyroid Association guidelines task force on thyroid nodules and differentiated thyroid cancer. Thyroid 2016;26:1–133.

32. Nanni C, Rubello D, Fanti S, et al. Role of 18F-FDG-PET and PET/CT imaging in thyroid cancer. Biomed Pharmacother 2006;60(8):409–13.

33. Ding W, Ruan G, Zhu J, et al. Metastatic site discriminates survival benefit of primary tumor surgery for differentiated thyroid cancer with distant metastases: a real-world observational study. Medicine (Baltimore) 2020;99(48):e23132.

34. Kim BS, Kim SJ, Kim IJ, et al. Factors associated with positive F-18 fluorodeoxyglucose positron emission tomography before thyroidectomy in patients with papillary thyroid carcinoma. Thyroid 2012;22:725–9.

35. Jeong HS, Baek CH, Son YI, et al. Integrated 18F-FDG PET/CT for the initial evaluation of cervical node level of patients with papillary thyroid carcinoma: comparison with ultrasound and contrast-enhanced CT. Clin Endocrinol 2006;65:402–7.

36. Choi WH, Chung YA, Han EJ, et al. Clinical value of integrated [18F]fluoro-2-deoxy-D-glucose positron emission tomography/computed tomography in the preoperative assessment of papillary thyroid carcinoma: comparison with sonography. J Ultrasound Med 2011;30:1267–73.

37. Morita S, Mizoguchi K, Suzuki M, et al. The accuracy of (18)[F]-fluoro-2-deoxy-D-glucose-positron emission tomography/computed tomography, ultrasonography, and enhanced computed tomography alone in the preoperative diagnosis of cervical lymph node metastasis in patients with papillary thyroid carcinoma. World J Surg 2010;34:2564–9.

38. Lee JW, Lee SM, Lee DH, et al. Clinical utility of 18F-FDG PET/CT concurrent with 131I therapy in intermediate-to-high-risk patients with differentiated thyroid cancer: dual-center experience with 286 patients. J Nucl Med 2013;54(8):1230–6.

39. Rosenbaum-Krumme SJ, Görges R, Bockisch A, et al. 18FFDG-PET/CT changes therapy management in high-risk DTC after first radioiodine therapy. Eur J Nucl Med Mol Imaging 2012;39:1373–80.

40. Ghossein R, Livolsi VA. Papillary thyroid carcinoma tall cell variant. Thyroid 2008;18(11):1179–81.

41. Kuo CS, Tang KT, Lin JD, et al. Diffuse sclerosing variant of papillary thyroid carcinoma with multiple metastases and elevated serum carcinoembryonic antigen level. Thyroid 2012;22(11):1187–90.

42. Xu YH, Song HJ, Qiu ZL, et al. Extensive lymph node metastases found by (18)F-FDG-PET/CT in a patient with a diffuse sclerosing variant of papillary thyroid carcinoma. Hellenic J Nucl Med 2011;14(2):188–9.

43. Wong TZ, Jain MK, Spratt SE. I-131, I-123, and F-18 FDG-PET imaging in a patient with a diffuse sclerosing variant of papillary thyroid cancer. Clin Nucl Med 2008;33(12):834–7.

44. Giovanella L, Fasolini F, Suriano S, et al. Hyperfunctioning solid/trabecular follicular carcinoma of the thyroid gland. J Oncol 2010;2010:635984.

45. Diehl M, Graichen S, Menzel C, et al. F-18 FDG PET in insular thyroid cancer. Clin Nucl Med 2003;28(9):728–31.

46. Leboulleux S, El Bez I, Borget I, et al. Post radioiodine treatment whole-body scan in the era of 18-fluorodeoxyglucose positron emission tomography for differentiated thyroid carcinoma with elevated serum thyroglobulin levels. Thyroid 2012;22:832–8.

47. Dong MJ, Liu ZF, Zhao K, et al. Value of 18F-FDG-PET/PET-CT in differentiated thyroid carcinoma with radioiodine-negative whole-body scan: a meta-analysis. Nucl Med Commun 2009;30:639–50.

48. Miller ME, Chen Q, Elashoff D, et al. Positron emission tomography and positron emission tomography-CT evaluation for recurrent papillary thyroid carcinoma: meta-analysis and literature review. Head Neck 2011;33:562–5.

49. Haslerud T, Brauckhoff K, Reisæter L, et al. F18-FDG-PET for recurrent differentiated thyroid cancer: a systematic meta-analysis. Acta Radiol 2016;57:1193–200.

50. Ma C, Xie J, Lou Y, et al. The role of TSH for 18F-FDG-PET in diagnosing recurrence and metastases of differentiated thyroid carcinoma with elevated Tg and negative scan: a meta-analysis. Eur J Endocrinol 2010;163:177–83.

51. Abraham T, Schöder H. Thyroid cancer–indications and opportunities for positron emission tomography/computed emission tomography/computed tomography imaging. Semin Nucl Med 2011;41:121–38.

52. Giovanella L, Ceriani L, De Palma D, et al. Relationship between serum Tg and 18FDG-PET/CT in 131I-negative differentiated thyroid carcinomas. Head Neck 2012;34:626–31.

53. Giovanella L, Trimboli P, Verburg FA, et al. Tg levels and Tg doubling time independently predict a positive (18) FFDG PET/CT scan in patients with biochemical recurrence of differentiated thyroid carcinoma. Eur J Nucl Med Mol Imaging 2013;40:874–80.

54. Kim SJ, Lee SW, Pak K, et al. Diagnostic performance of PET in thyroid cancer with elevated anti-Tg-ab. Endocr Relat Cancer 2018;25:643–52.

55. Robbins R, Wan Q, Grewal R, et al. Real-time prognosis for metastatic thyroid carcinoma based on 2-[18F]fluoro-2-deoxy-D-glucose-positron emission tomography scanning. J Clin Endocrinol Metab 2006;91:498–505.

56. Schönberger J, Rüschoff J, Grimm D, et al. Glucose transporter1 gene expression is related to thyroid neoplasms with an unfavorable prognosis: an immunohistochemical study. Thyroid 2002;12:747–54.

57. Nagamachi S, Wakamatsu H, Kiyohara S, et al. Comparison of diagnostic and prognostic capabilities of 18F-FDG-PET/CT, 131I-scintigraphy, and diffusion-weighted magnetic resonance imaging for postoperative thyroid cancer. Jpn J Radiol 2011;29:413–22.

58. Deandreis D, Al Ghuzlan A, Leboulleux S, et al. Do histological, immunohistochemical, and metabolic (radioiodine and fluorodeoxyglucose uptakes) patterns of metastatic thyroid cancer correlate with the patient outcome? Endocr Relat Cancer 2011;13(18):159–69.

59. Vural GU, Akkas BE, Ercakmak N, et al. Prognostic significance of FDG PET/CT on the follow-up of patients of differentiated thyroid carcinoma with negative 131I whole-body scan and elevated Tg levels: correlation with clinical and histopathologic characteristics and long-term follow-up data. Clin Nucl Med 2012;37:953–9.

60. Marcus C, Antoniou A, Rahmim A, et al. Fluorodeoxyglucose positron emission tomography/computerized tomography in differentiated thyroid cancer management: the importance of clinical justification and value in predicting survival. J Med Imaging Radiatoncol 2015;59:281–8.

61. Bogsrud TV, Hay ID, Karantanis D, et al. Prognostic value of 18Ffluorodeoxyglucose-positron emission tomography in patients with differentiated thyroid carcinoma and circulating anti Tg autoantibodies. Nucl Med Commun 2011;32:245–51.

62. Santhanam P, Khthir R, Solnes LB, et al. The relationship of BRAF(V600E) mutation status to FDG PET/CT avidity in thyroid cancer: a review and meta-analysis. Endocr Pract 2018;24:21–6.

63. Iwano S, Kato K, Ito S, et al. FDG PET performed concurrently with initial I-131 ablation for differentiated thyroid cancer. Ann Nucl Med 2012;26:207–13.

64. Piccardo A, Foppiani L, Morbelli S, et al. Could [18] F-fluorodeoxyglucose PET/CT changed the therapeutic management of stage IV thyroid cancer with positive (131) I whole body scan? Q J Nucl Med Mol Imaging 2011;55:57–65.

65. Haugen BR, Sherman SI. Evolving approaches to patients with advanced differentiated thyroid cancer. Endocr Rev 2013;34:439–55.

66. Baudin E, Schlumberger M. New therapeutic approaches for metastatic thyroid carcinoma. Lancet Oncol 2007;8:148–56.

67. Marotta V, Ramundo V, Camera L, et al. Sorafenib in advanced iodine-refractory differentiated thyroid cancer: efficacy, safety and exploratory analysis of the role of serum Tg and FDG-PET. Clin Endocrinol 2013;78:760–7.

68. Carr LL, Mankoff DA, Goulart BH, et al. Phase II, the study of daily Sunitinib in FDG-PET-positive, iodine-refractory differentiated thyroid cancer and metastatic medullary carcinoma of the thyroid with functional imaging correlation. Clin Cancer Res 2010;16:5260–8.

69. Ahmaddy F, Burgard C, Beyer L, et al. 18F-FDG-PET/CT in patients with advanced, radioiodine refractory thyroid cancer treated with lenvatinib. Cancers (Basel) 2021;13(2):317.

70. Ahlman H, Tisell LE, Wangberg B, et al. The relevance of somatostatin receptors in thyroid neoplasia. Yale J Biol Med 1997;70:523–33.

71. Ain KB, Taylor KD, Tofiq S, et al. Somatostatin receptor subtype expression in human thyroid and thyroid carcinoma cell lines. J Clin Endocrinol Metab 1997;82:1857–62.

72. Kundu P, Lata S, Sharma P, et al. Prospective evaluation of 68Ga-DOTANOC PET-CT in differentiated

thyroid cancer patients with raised thyroglobulin and negative 131Iwhole-body scan: comparison with 18F-FDG PET-CT. Eur J Nucl Med Mol Imaging 2014;41:1354–62.

73. Middendorp M, Selkinski I, Happel C, et al. Comparison of positron emission tomography with [18F]FDG and [68Ga]DOTATOC in recurrent differentiated thyroid cancer: preliminary data. Q J Nucl Med Mol Imaging 2010;54:76–83.

74. Traub-Weidinger T, Putzer D, von Guggenberg E, et al. Multiparametric PET im-aging in thyroid malignancy characterizing tumour heterogeneity: somatostatin receptors and glucose metabolism. Eur J Nucl Med Mol Imaging 2015;42:1995–2001.

75. Versari A, Sollini M, Frasoldati A, et al. Differentiated thyroid cancer: a new perspective with radiolabeled somatostatin analogues for imaging and treatment of patients. Thyroid 2014;24:715–26.

76. Parihar AS, Mittal BR, Kumar R, et al. 68Ga-DOTA-RGD2 positron emission tomography/computed tomography in radioiodine refractory thyroid cancer: prospective comparison of diagnostic accuracy with 18 F-FDG positron emission tomography/computed tomography and evaluation toward potential theranostics. Thyroid 2020;30(4):557–67.

77. Ballal S, Yadav MP, Gupta AK, et al. Comparison of conventional ultrasound, Doppler, elastography, and contrast-enhanced ultrasonography parameters with histology findings in the differential diagnosis of benign and malignant thyroid nodules. Thyroid Disord Ther 2017;6:2.

78. Freudenberg LS, Antoch G, Jentzen W, et al. Value of (124)I-PET/CT in staging of patients with differentiated thyroid cancer. Eur Radiol 2004;14:2092–8.

79. Freudenberg LS, Jentzen W, Stahl A, et al. Clinical applications of 124I-PET/CT in patients with differentiated thyroid cancer. Eur J Nucl Med Mol Imaging 2011;38:S48–56.

80. Van Nostrand D, Moreau S, Bandaru VV, et al. 124)I positron emission tomography versus (131)I planar imaging in the identification of residual thyroid tissue and/or metastasis in patients who have well-differentiated thyroid cancer. Thyroid 2010;20:879–83.

81. Capoccetti F, Criscuoli B, Rossi G, et al. The effectiveness of 124I PET/CT in patients with differentiated thyroid cancer. Q J Nucl Med Mol Imaging 2009;53:536–45.

82. Khorjekar GR, Van Nostrand D, Garcia C, et al. Do negative 124I pretherapy positron emission tomography scans in patients with elevated serum thyroglobulin levels predict negative 131I posttherapy scans? Thyroid 2014;24:1394–9.

83. De Pont C, Halders S, Bucerius J, et al. 124-I PET/CT in the pretherapeutic staging of differentiated thyroid carcinoma: comparison with posttherapy 131I SPECT/CT. Eur J Nucl Med Mol Imaging 2013;40:693–700.

84. Ruhlmann M, Jentzen W, Ruhlmann V, et al. High level of agreement between pretherapeutic 124I PET and intratherapeutic 131I imaging in detecting iodine-positive thyroid cancer metastases. J Nucl Med 2016;57:1339–42.

85. Stojadinovic A, Ghossein RA, Hoos A, et al. Hürthle cell carcinoma: a critical histopathologic appraisal. J Clin Oncol 2001;19:2616–25.

86. Pryma DA, Schöder H, Gönen M, et al. Diagnostic accuracy and prognostic value of 18F-FDG PET in Hürthle cell thyroid cancer patients. J Nucl Med 2006;47(8):1260–6.

87. Nikiforov YE. Genetic alterations involved in the transition from well-differentiated to poorly differentiated and anaplastic thyroid carcinomas. Endocr Pathol 2004;15(4):319–27.

88. Treglia G, Muoio B, Giovanella L, et al. The role of positron emission tomography and positron emission tomography/computed tomography in thyroid tumours: an overview. Eur Arch Otorhinolaryngol 2013;270(6):1783–7.

89. Grabellus F, Nagarajah J, Bockisch A, et al. Glucose transporter1 expression, tumor proliferation, and iodine/glucose uptake in thyroid cancer with emphasis on poorly differentiated thyroid carcinoma. Clin Nucl Med 2012;37(2):121–7.

90. Kim CH, Yoole R, Chung YA, et al. Influence of thyroid-stimulating hormone on 18F-fluorodeoxyglucose and 99mTc-methoxyisobutylisonitrile uptake in human poorly differentiated thyroid cancer cells in vitro. Ann Nucl Med 2009;23(2):131–6.

91. Are C, Shaha AR. Anaplastic thyroid carcinoma: biology, pathogenesis, prognostic factors, and treatment approaches. Ann Surg Oncol 2006; 13(4):453–64.

92. Chiacchio S, Lorenzoni A, Boni G, et al. Anaplastic thyroid cancer: prevalence, diagnosis, and treatment. Minerva Endocrinol 2008;33(4):341–57.

93. Smallridge RC, Ain KB, Asa SL, et al. American thyroid association anaplastic thyroid cancer guidelines Taskforce. American thyroid association guidelines for the management of patients with anaplastic thyroid cancer. Thyroid 2012;22(11): 1104–39.

94. Poisson T, Deandreis D, Leboulleux S, et al. 18F-fluorodeoxyglucose positron emission tomography and computed tomography in anaplastic thyroid cancer. Eur J Nucl Med Mol Imaging 2010;37(12): 2277–85.

95. Bogsrud TV, Karantanis D, Nathan MA, et al. 18F-FDG PET in the management of patients with anaplastic thyroid carcinoma. Thyroid 2008;18(7): 713–9.

96. Trimboli P, Giovanella L, Crescenzi A, et al. Medullary thyroid cancer diagnosis: an appraisal. Head Neck 2014;36:1216–23.

97. Wells SA Jr, Asa SL, Dralle H, et al. Revised American Thyroid Association guidelines for the management of medullary thyroid carcinoma. Thyroid 2015;25:567–610.

98. Rubello D, Rampin L, Nanni C, et al. The role of 18F-FDG PET/CT in detecting metastatic deposits of recurrent medullary thyroid carcinoma: a prospective study. Eur J Surg Oncol 2008;34(5):581–6.

99. Oudoux A, Salaun PY, Bournaud C, et al. Sensitivity and prognostic value of positron emission tomography with F-18-fluorodeoxyglucose and sensitivity of immunoscintigraphy in patients with medullary thyroid carcinoma treated with anticarcinoembryonic antigen-targeted radioimmunotherapy. J Clin Endocrinol Metab 2007;92(12):4590–7.

100. Treglia G, Rufini V, Salvatori M, et al. PET imaging in recurrent medullary thyroid carcinoma. Int J Mol Imaging 2012;2012:324686.

101. Rufini V, Treglia G, Perotti G, et al. Role of PET in medullary thyroid carcinoma. Minerva Endocrinol 2008;33:67–73.

102. Slavikova K, Montravers F, Treglia G, et al. What is currently the best radiopharmaceutical for the hybrid PET/CT detection of recurrent medullary thyroid carcinoma? CurrRadiopharm 2013;6:96–105.

103. Treglia G, Stefanelli A, Castaldi P, et al. A standardized dual-phase 18F-DOPA PET/CT protocol in the detection of medullary thyroid cancer. Nucl Med Commun 2013;34:185–6.

104. Treglia G, Tamburello A, Giovanella L. Detection rate of somatostatin receptor PET in patients with recurrent medullary thyroid carcinoma: a systematic review and a meta-analysis. Hormones (Athens) 2017;16(4):262–72.

105. Romero-Lluch AR, Cuenca-Cuenca JI, Guerrero-Vázquez R, et al. Diagnostic utility of PET/CT with (18)F-DOPA and (18)F-FDG in persistent or recurrent medullary thyroid carcinoma: the importance of calcitonin and carcinoembryonic antigen cutoff. Eur J Nucl Med Mol Imaging 2017;44(12):2004–13.

106. Ansell SM, Grant CS, Habermann TM. Primary thyroid lymphoma. Semin Oncol 1999;26:316–23.

107. Basu S, Li G, Bural G, et al. Fluorodeoxyglucose positron emission tomography (FDG-PET) and PET/computed tomography imaging characteristics of thyroid lymphoma and their potential clinical utility. Acta Radiol 2009;50(2):201–4.

108. Damle NA, Bal CS, Singh TP, et al. Anaplastic thyroid carcinoma on 68 Ga-PSMA PET/CT: opening new frontiers. Eur J Nucl Med Mol Imaging 2018;45(4):667–8.

109. Heitkötter B, Steinestel K, Trautmann M, et al. Neovascular PSMA expression is a common feature in malignant neoplasms of the thyroid. Oncotarget 2018;9(11):9867–74.

110. Bodet-Milin C, Faivre-Chauvet A, Carlier T, et al. Immuno-PET using anticarcinoembryonic antigen bispecific antibody and 68Ga-labeled peptide in metastatic medullary thyroid carcinoma: clinical optimization of the Pretargeting parameters in a first-in-human trial. J Nucl Med 2016;57(10):1505–11.

111. Ong SC, Schöder H, Patel SG, et al. Diagnostic accuracy of 18F-FDG PET in re-staging patients with medullary thyroid carcinoma and elevated calcitonin levels. J Nucl Med 2007;48(4):501–7.

112. Fu H, Fu J, Huang J, et al. 68Ga-FAPI PET/CT in thyroid cancer with thyroglobulin elevation and negative iodine scintigraphy. Clin Nucl Med 2021;46(5):427–30.

PET/CT: Nasopharyngeal Cancers

Chenyi Xie, MBBS, Varut Vardhanabhuti, MBBS, FRCR, PhD*

KEYWORDS

• PET • Nasopharyngeal cancers • Staging • Diagnostic imaging

KEY POINTS

- PET imaging provides value in the diagnostic work-up with strengths in N and M staging as well as treatment planning.
- Novel quantitative techniques are increasingly used and may provide valuable prognostic information.
- Potential pitfall in false-positive must be borne in mind in the context of posttreatment change which is outlined in this article.

INTRODUCTION

Nasopharyngeal carcinoma (NPC) is the predominant tumor type arising from the mucosal lining of the nasopharynx, the tubular passage behind the nasal cavity which connects the oropharynx below. The histologic distinction is different to most other head and neck cancers which often are squamous cell carcinomas. The GLOBOCAN 2018 reported 129,079 new cases and 72,987 deaths of NPC worldwide.[1] NPC is distinct for its unbalanced geographic distribution. It is highly prevalent in Southeast Asia and Southern China whereby approximately 70% of the newly diagnosed cases were made.[2,3] It is rare in the United States and Western Europe, with an incidence of only 0.5 to 2 cases per 100,000. In Southern China, the disease is more prevalent and the annual incidence rate could reach 11.6 per 100,000 person-years in the high incidence areas.[3–6] To date, there have been improvements in the management of NPC. The incidence rate for NPC is decreasing gradually and the underlying reason could be reduced tobacco consumptions, changed dietary patterns, and economic growth.[7] Although the overall survival for patients with NPC has been improving with a number of recent advances in treatment technologies, locally advanced disease is still frequently encountered with 70% of newly diagnosed patients with NPC being at locally advanced stages at the time of diagnosis.[8,9]

CLINICAL PRESENTATION

NPC frequently originates from the pharyngeal recess, the fossa of Rosenmüller. As this is a clinically occult site, patients may remain asymptomatic for a prolonged period adding to the difficulty in diagnosis. The most common presenting complaints are headache, diplopia, or facial numbness, caused by cranial nerve involvement due to the erosion of skull base, and a mass in the neck, due to cervical node metastases. Other symptoms include nasal obstruction with epistaxis, and serous otitis media which may occur infrequently, but if present usually indicates locally advanced disease. There is a tendency for early metastatic spread with lymph node metastases being present at diagnosis in 75 to 90% of cases and are bilateral in over 50%. Distant metastases are present at diagnosis in 5 to 11% of patients with the most frequent sites being bone, lung, and liver.

NORMAL ANATOMY OF NASOPHARYNX REGION

Nasopharynx, as the upmost part of the pharynx, lies below the central base of the skull and above

Department of Diagnostic Radiology, Li Ka Shing Faculty of Medicine, University of Hong Kong, K406, Block K, Queen Mary Hospital, Pokfulam Road, Hong Kong SAR, China
* Corresponding author.
E-mail address: varv@hku.hk

PET Clin 17 (2022) 285–296
https://doi.org/10.1016/j.cpet.2021.12.006
1556-8598/22/© 2021 Elsevier Inc. All rights reserved.

pet.theclinics.com

the level of the free border of the soft palate. The anatomy of the nasopharyngeal area is complex. It neighbors anteriorly the air-containing nasal cavity via the posterior nasal apertures (choanae). The posterior aspect of the nasopharynx is bounded by the clivus, prevertebral musculatures, and the C1 and C2 cervical vertebrae and the pharyngeal tonsil (adenoids) lie in this area. On its lateral wall is the pharyngeal orifice of the Eustachian tube connecting the torus tubaris and the fossae of Rosenmuller (posterolateral pharyngeal recess).[10,11] The fossae of Rosenmuller are common sites of origin of nasopharyngeal cancers.[3] The nasopharyngeal area has 2 lymphatic drainages.[12,13] One goes laterally along the pharyngeal wall piercing the superior musculatures into the lateral retropharyngeal and cervical lymph nodes (both jugular and spinal accessory chains). The other one runs along the posterior wall of the pharyngeal area from the visceral fascia at the roof to the medial retropharyngeal lymph nodes. Enlarged retropharyngeal lymph node should, therefore, prompt investigation for NPC even if the primary tumor is not obvious.

IMAGING TECHNIQUE

The most commonly used imaging modalities for the staging and radiotherapy planning of NPC include magnetic resonance imaging (MRI), computed tomography (CT), and [18F]-fluorodeoxyglucose (FDG) positron emission tomography/CT (PET/CT). MR imaging is a preferred choice for the assessment of the primary tumor of NPC for its high-resolution determination of soft tissue manifestations.[14] Contrast-enhanced CT provides an alternative assessment of lymph node metastasis.[15,16] But the sensitivity of CT imaging alone is not satisfactory. PET/CT could offer additional physiologic information over CT/MR imaging and is being increasingly used for the clinical staging classification. Currently, the 18F-FDG is the most commonly used radiotracer for PET imaging in patients with NPC. FDG could aid in the assessment of metabolic function targeted regions. However, FDG is not a tumour-specific tracer. Uptake of 18F-FDG in benign nonphysiologic lesions could be observed in greater than 25% of the PET/CT scans for patients with confirmed or suspected cancers.[17]

IMAGING FINDINGS/PATHOLOGY

Nasopharyngeal tumors are hypermetabolic on PET imaging. At diagnosis, these can be large and bulky, and can be locally invasive around the surrounding structures (Fig. 1). Although MR imaging has better soft tissue differentiation, the

value of PET in primary tumor assessment may be to add more confidence in delineating the extent of tumor involvement compared with surrounding edematous change.

In the assessment of nodal spread, the route is usually via the retropharyngeal region and then to the cervical region. Sometimes the primary tumor and retropharyngeal nodal disease are not separable (see Fig. 1B). Small nodes based on the size on CT could be reactive or due to early metastatic deposit. Increased metabolic activity even in small lymph nodes can increase confidence in the diagnosis of early nodal spread (Fig. 2). With the added information of CT, invasion of the adjacent bone (such as the clivus) can also be more confidently assessed (Fig. 3).

The main indication for using PET-CT imaging is for the assessment of metastatic disease which can occur more commonly with locally advanced primary tumor (eg, see Fig. 4). Metastases can occur in the lung, liver, and bones (Fig. 5).

CLINICAL APPLICATIONS AND DIAGNOSTIC CRITERIA
Staging

Definitive diagnosis is made with endoscope-guided biopsy of the primary tumor. Imaging is often performed after initial histologic confirmation. The current staging system is mainly based on the recently updated International Union Against Cancer (UICC) and the American Joint Committee on Cancer (AJCC) TNM Classification criteria (eighth edition, 2016).[18,19]

T Staging

With better soft-tissue visualization than CT, MR imaging is currently a superior choice for a more accurate assessment of the primary tumor site(s), deep tumoural infiltration, and retropharyngeal lymph node involvement at an early stage.[8,20,21] PET/CT could offer an acceptable diagnostic value but was less sensitive than MR imaging in finding subtle abnormalities in the intracranial area, parapharyngeal space, skull base, and sphenoid sinus, which may result in T stage downstaging.[22] Some studies reported that functional MR imaging could provide additional biological information. The intravoxel incoherent motion characteristics collected from diffusion-weighted MR imaging are shown to be predictors for pretreatment staging[23] and for posttreatment assessment between recurrence and fibrosis in the skull base of patients with NPC.[24] Similar to MR imaging, PET could provide some functional parameters. Enhanced diagnostic performance of FDG PET/CT in NPC was shown with the use of some conventional

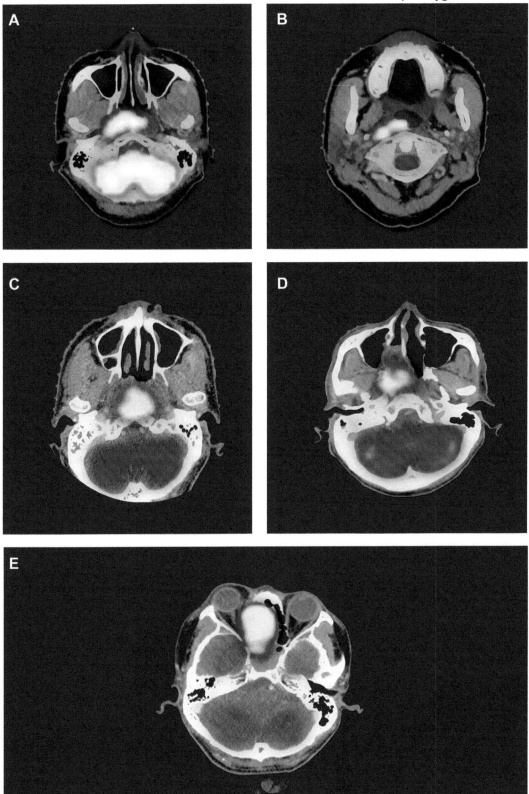

Fig. 1. (*A*, *B*) Fused PET-CT image of primary NPC showing markedly hypermetabolic tumor in the nasopharynx. Note that it is not uncommon for the primary tumor and the retropharyngeal to appear to be inseparable as this is a common drainage site. (*C*) Another example of bulky markedly hypermetabolic primary NPC tumor. (*D*) and (*E*) More examples of bulky markedly hypermetabolic primary NPC tumor which can be locally invasive with involvement of the nasal cavity.

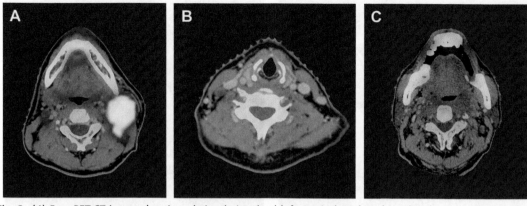

Fig. 2. (*A*) Fuse PET-CT image showing obviously involved left cervical IIA lymph node. The contralateral small right cervical IIA lymph node also demonstrates mild increased metabolic activity. Nodal metastasis has to be suspected in this case. (*B*) A mildly hypermetabolic mildly enlarged right cervical IV lymph node is noted. Increased metabolic activity raises confidence in the diagnosis of malignant spread. (*C*) Another example mildly hypermetabolic cervical lymph node demonstrating the value of PET in diagnosis nodal metastasis.

quantitative features, such as standardized uptake value (SUV), tumor volume, and total lesion glycolysis (TLG). TLG of the primary tumor is reported to be significantly correlated with tumor burden and tumor staging.[25]

N Staging

PET/CT is reported to be better for the detection of small-size cervical lymph nodes.[3,20,26] Peng and colleagues[26] demonstrated that compared with MR imaging, PET/CT was a better diagnostic tool for small cervical lymph nodes (≥ 5 and <10 mm diameters), which contributed to a more precise clinical staging. Improvement in accuracy of PET in detecting metastatic lymph nodes compared with MR imaging was also confirmed by correlation with histopathology, which demonstrated a diagnostic accuracy, sensitivity, and specificity of 89.2%, 94.1%, and 85.0% for 18F-FDG PET/CT, respectively.[27] Functional parameters in PET like SUVmax in lymph nodes have been reported to be a prognostic factor for patients with NPC.[28,29]

Some retropharyngeal lymph nodes might be missed on PET/CT images because these lymph nodes are close to the primary tumor sites.[30] Therefore, some studies have examined the clinical utility of performing PET-MR imaging. PET/MR imaging was particularly useful for distinguishing retropharyngeal nodal metastasis from adjacent nasopharyngeal tumors.[31] Regarding the N staging assessment, the sensitivity of PET/MR imaging (99.5%) was higher than that of head and neck MR imaging (94.2%) and PET/CT (90.9%). Given the high cost of PET-MR imaging, cost-effectiveness needs to be borne in mind and more studies are needed to ascertain the benefit in this regard.

M Staging

PET/CT is reported to be better for the staging of distant metastasis than conventional work-up (eg, chest/abdomen/pelvis CT scan and bone scan), and is also preferred in high-risk patients for recurrence disease evaluation.[3,20,22,32]

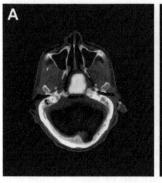
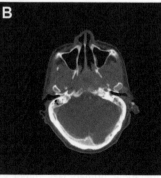

Fig. 3. (*A*) PET-CT fused image and (*B*) CT showing primary NPC tumor with clivus bone destruction. The blooming effect that can be seen with PET activity can sometimes make it difficult to be confident if there is adjacent bone destruction. In this case, the corresponding CT viewed in bone window increases confidence in this diagnosis demonstrating destructive bony changes.

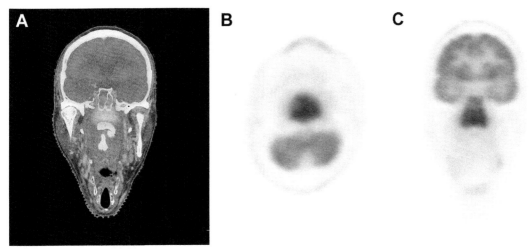

Fig. 4. (*A–C*) Bulky primary tumor with skull base invasion (*A*) coronal postcontrast CT, (*B*) axial PET, and (*C*) coronal PET images.

Ng and colleagues[22] reported a significantly higher sensitivity of PET/CT (81.3%) for detecting distant metastasis than that of conventional work-up (25.0%). As the physiologic uptake of the brain region is high, and relatively lower image resolution, PET/CT is also not an ideal tool for the evaluation of intracranial disease.[33] Recently, PET/MR images were shown to be more accurate than PET/CT images for mapping intracranial invasion.[31]

Treatment Planning

With the advent of IMRT, it has become of paramount importance to accurately delineate gross tumor volume (GTV) for irradiation. To this end, it has been shown that PET improves tumor and lymph node delineation for treatment with IMRT[27,34,35] with survival benefit in locally advanced disease. For example, in locoregional advanced patients with NPC staged III-IVB, compared with CT-based IMRT, FDG-PET/CT-guided dose painting-IMRT significantly improved 3-year local failure-free survival (LFFS, 98.8% vs 91.3%; $P = .032$), locoregional failure-free survival (LRFFS, 97.2 vs 91.2%; $P = .049$), distant metastasis-free survival (DMFS, 92.9% vs 87.4%; $P = .041$), disease-free survival (DFS, 87.9% vs 82.4%; $P = .02$), and overall survival (OS, 91.8% vs 82.6%; $P = .049$).[34]

Posttreatment Imaging

In addition to staging, imaging has been used for detecting recurrence. PET is superior in detecting nodal malignancy but has limitations in the accurate assessment of lymph node size because of poor anatomic resolution. CT can provide better measurement for lymph node size and anatomic information. The combination of multiple imaging modalities (eg, PET/CT) could significantly improve the diagnostic accuracy.[36] SUVmax in primary tumor site(s) has been shown to be prognostic for patients with NPC.[28,37] Posttreatment PET/CT could improve the diagnostic sensitivity and specificity for local residual or recurrent cancers.[38] A meta-analysis by Wei and colleagues[39] showed that the combined specificity for PET/CT was significantly better than MR imaging (93% vs 76%). However, inflammation lesions introduced by radiotherapy and chemotherapy could confound the identification of local residual, recurrent NPC, or regional lymph node involvement. CT has the ability to depict abnormal anatomic changes and PET can further provide FDG metabolic uptake information in the lesions. Typically, tumor recurrence seems hypermetabolic whereas posttreatment chronic fibrosis usually does not demonstrate uptake.[38] In the short-term posttreatment period, whereby there may still be some inflammatory reaction, these areas can seem hypermetabolic, and may further confound interpretation. Usually, this should resolve within 3 months after treatment cessation. The fused imaging modalities help to directly assess the anatomic structures and biological functions spontaneously, which reduces the false-positive rate. Furthermore, follow-up scans are suggested for better differentiation of posttreatment inflammation and malignant diseases.[40,41]

Osteoradionecrosis is radiation-induced bone necrosis that may occur as early as 1 year after treatment. This is associated with a slow healing process, and often with surrounding inflammatory changes. Differentiating this from tumor recurrence or osteomyelitis can be difficult, as areas of osteoradionecrosis could appear with FDG

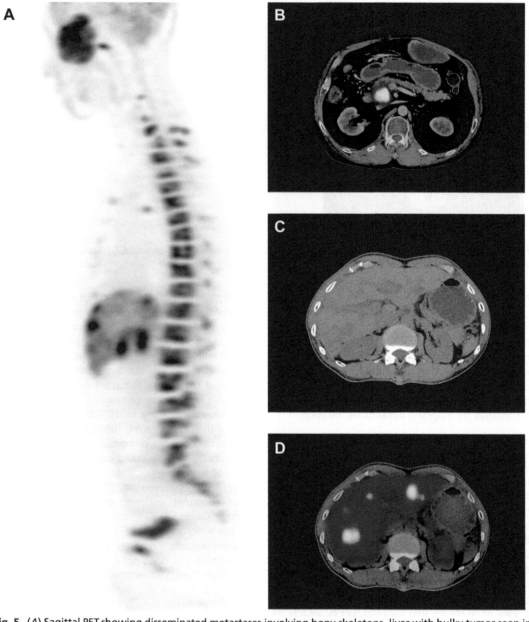

Fig. 5. (*A*) Sagittal PET showing disseminated metastases involving bony skeletons, liver with bulky tumor seen in the nasopharynx. (*B*) Axial fused PET-CT image showing enlarged/hypermetabolic abdominal lymph node metastasis. (*C*) CT and (*D*) fused PET-CT showing several hypodense/hypermetabolic liver metastases.

uptake in PET imaging.[42,43] Some CT and MR imaging features have been shown to be helpful for the determination of osteoradionecrosis.[44,45] Multi-modality imaging is preferred in high-risk patients for recurrence disease evaluation. If there is any diagnostic uncertainty, then histologic correlation is recommended.

Posttreatment condition such as temporal lobe necrosis has been known to occur in patients with NPC posttherapy in late stage, as NPC frequently invades skull base, and it may be inevitable that the temporal lobes are included in the radiation field. Distinguishing changes seen in the temporal lobe can sometimes be problematic. PET scan has been used in the context of differentiating radiation-induced necrosis (with the area appearing hypometabolic) from recurrent tumor (with the area appearing hypermetabolic), and have demonstrated reasonable differentiating capability,[46] but collaborative imaging (eg,

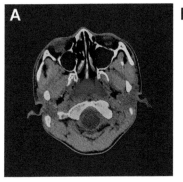
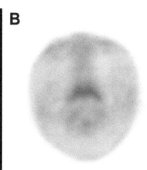

Fig. 6. A normal nasopharynx appearance in a young patient (A) fused PET-CT image and (B) axial PET image of the nasopharyngeal region.

functional MR imaging) may be helpful to reduce false-positive rate.[47]

DIFFERENTIAL DIAGNOSIS

The main differential diagnosis for a hypermetabolic nasopharyngeal lesion is nasopharyngeal lymphoma. Of note, the NK T-cell lymphoma is a particular subtype that affects the nasal cavity and may extend toward the nasopharyngeal region. Other conditions that may mimic nasopharyngeal tumors may include infection and inflammation, but usually, the diagnosis should be obvious from clinical history and findings. In such cases, there is often no need for dedicated imaging. Occasionally, inflammatory pseudotumour lesions may be encountered and these are often indistinguishable radiologically from tumors and will require histologic confirmation. For other tumoural lesions, lesions such as juvenile nasopharyngeal angiofibroma may seem hypermetabolic on PET, but these have distinct appearances being very vascular and also occur predominantly in children and adolescents. Malignant lesions such as rhabdomyosarcoma are also hypermetabolic on PET and have a bimodal distribution in children occurring in patients aged 2 to 4 years and 12 to 16 years. Age is an important discrimination factor and when children or young adults present with a mass in this region, these differential diagnoses must be borne in mind.

In young patients, there is often a symmetric fullness appearance in the nasopharyngeal region and may seem mildly hypermetabolic on PET (Fig. 6). Normally mild to moderate metabolic activity could be observed in some normal lymphatic tissues because 18F-FDG might accumulate in lymphocytes and macrophage cells.[48] The lymphatic tissues of the Waldeyer's ring could often confound the diagnosis of NPC. More comprehensive examination using CT, MR imaging, or invasive endoscopy could be adopted for accurate interpretation of suspected diseases.[49,50] Occasionally, inflammation is reported to be one of the most common causes for increased FDG uptake in benign lesions for PET/CT scans.[17]

ADVANCED TECHNIQUES

In current clinical practice, radiologists evaluate tumor diseases mainly by some qualitative features, which are also called semantic features. These observed radiological traits include a description of the tumoural border, regularity of margins, density, and heterogeneous

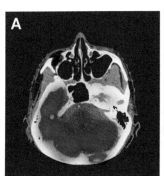
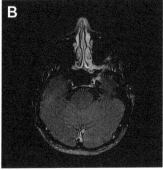

Fig. 7. PostchemoRT assessment. (A) Axial fused PET-CT image and (B) axial MR imaging T1W postcontrast image showing subtle mild hypermetabolic activity in a slightly expanded left pterygo-palatine fossa. In the corresponding MR imaging this shows mild soft tissue enhancement. Appearances are thought to represent residual disease. It must be noted that this may be difficult to differentiate from posttreatment change.

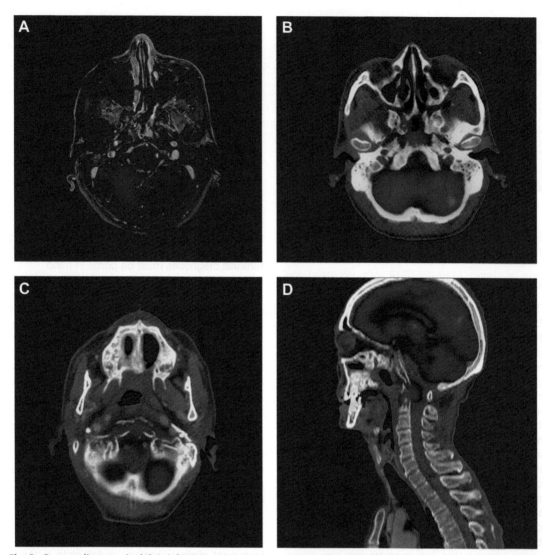

Fig. 8. Osteoradionecrosis. (*A*) Axial MR imaging T1W postcontrast image with irregularly enhancing mass at the posterior nasopharynx involving the clivus and (*B*) corresponding axial fused PET-CT image showing destructive lesion at the clivus, with increased metabolic activity. (*C*) Axial fused PET-CT image and (*D*) sagittal fused PET-CT image demonstrating areas of destruction involving C2 vertebra with hypermetabolism and associated soft tissue mass which extends posteriorly in the spinal canal. In this context, it may be difficult to differentiate from recurrence. The lesion was biopsied and was shown to be chronic granulation tissues only with no malignant cells detected.

enhancement following the administration of contrast as well as anatomic relationships with neighboring structures. However, the identification of semantic features is mainly based on the visual assessment by experienced radiologists. These features are often qualitative in nature which may fail to provide a sufficient description of tumoural heterogeneity. Conventional quantitative features have been shown to be diagnostic and prognostic in NPC.[25,28,29,37] More subtle tumor characteristics could be captured by these continuously scaled measurements. Recently, with the rapid

development of technology, artificial intelligence (AI) methodologies have attracted much attention. First, radiomics have rapidly emerged as a possible discipline for tumor profiling in the medical imaging area.[51] High-dimensional radiomic features could be extracted directly from current imaging modalities with the employment of advanced imaging features extraction.[52] For example, compared with conventional metrics, the PET/CT radiomic-based model showed higher diagnostic value for posttreatment differentiation between recurrence and inflammation: in patients with NPC in terms of area under the receiver operating characteristic curve (AUC) values (0.867–0.892 vs 0.817).[53] Differentiation between NPC and chronic nasopharyngitis was also explored, and features robustness was found to be unrelated to final diagnostic performance.[54] Radiomics features extracted from PET-CT could also aid in prognostic tasks.[55–58] More recently, deep learning has been shown to provide useful information for clinical decision-making. The combination of deep learning features and radiomics has shown improved prognosis prediction for patients with NPC.[59] Traditional manual delineation of regions of interest requires laborious and time-consuming work from experienced radiologists. Automatic deep learning-based segmentation methods have shown potential for assistance during radiation planning.[60] The current findings have also proved the potential of AI approaches for clinical decision support systems.

CASE STUDY PRESENTATION
Case 1

A 52-year-old man initially presented with locally advanced NPC with the invasion of the skull base with T4N2M0 disease at staging. The patient had 3 cycles of induction chemoradiotherapy. A PET/CT scan was performed to assess the initial response. On the PET/CT, there is expansion of the left pterygopalatine fissure, associated with residual mild increased metabolic activity (**Fig. 7**A). A corresponding MR imaging is also shown (**Fig 7**B) with mild enhancement in these areas. This case illustrates the difficulty in distinguishing residual disease compared with posttreatment change. In this case, given that there was still some residual enhancing tissue on MR imaging and mildly hypermetabolic area on the PET image, it was thought that there was residual disease. The patient was treated with more cycles of chemotherapy, and after treatment completion, the metabolic activity resolved. Postbiopsy of nasopharynx was negative for malignant cells, and EBV DNA was 0 copies.

Case 2

A 63-year-old male patient with previous NPC was treated with chemoradiotherapy and remains in remission.

An irregular enhancing mass is noted in the MR imaging image (**Fig 8**A), with mild increased metabolic activity on PET (**Fig 8**B). This case illustrates the difficulty of distinguishing changes of osteonecrosis from tumor recurrence. The imaging findings can be nonspecific and is related to ongoing inflammatory changes. It is not uncommon to have to rely on histologic correlation for a definitive diagnosis. If there is any doubt regarding the diagnosis, then a biopsy should be recommended. More examples for another patient are shown in **Fig. 8**C, D. This can be associated with significant soft tissue mass, which in this case encroaches on the spinal canal posteriorly.

CONCLUSION/SUMMARY

PET/CT scan has been used as a tool for the diagnosis and management of NPC. It has been proven to be highly valuable for the imaging and management of these patients and is recommended to be incorporated in the standard clinical assessment workflow. MR imaging and PET have a complimentary role at staging with MR imaging playing a significant role in the assessment of primary tumor (T staging) and FDG PET having greater efficacy for N and M staging. The growing use of PET is also seen in treatment planning, with particular benefit in patient survival has been shown from using PET for the delineation of GTV in locally advanced diseases. Novel techniques such as the use of radiomics have been shown to provide valuable prognostic information. Increasing utilization of PET/MR imaging has been observed for a complete assessment at staging with the additional benefit of superior soft-tissue characterization, and the assessment of intracranial disease involvement.

CLINICS CARE POINTS

- PET imaging provides value in the diagnostic work-up with strengths in N and M staging as well as treatment planning.
- Novel quantitative techniques are increasingly used and may provide valuable prognostic information
- Potential pitfall in false-positive must be borne in mind in the context of posttreatment change which is outlined in this article.

DISCLOSURE

The authors have nothing to disclose.

REFERENCES

1. Bray F, Ferlay J, Soerjomataram I, et al. Global cancer statistics 2018: GLOBOCAN estimates of incidence and mortality worldwide for 36 cancers in

185 countries. CA Cancer J Clin 2018;68(6): 394–424.

2. Ferlay J, Ervik M, Lam F, et al. Global cancer observatory: cancer today. Lyon, France: International Agency for Research on Cancer; 2018.

3. Chen YP, Chan ATC, Le QT, et al. Nasopharyngeal carcinoma. Lancet (London, England) 2019; 394(10192):64–80.

4. Cao SM, Simons MJ, Qian CN. The prevalence and prevention of nasopharyngeal carcinoma in China. Chin J Cancer 2011;30(2):114–9.

5. Yu MC, Yuan JM. Epidemiology of nasopharyngeal carcinoma. Semin Cancer Biol 2002;12(6): 421–9.

6. Wei KR, Zheng RS, Zhang SW, et al. Nasopharyngeal carcinoma incidence and mortality in China, 2013. Chin J Cancer 2017;36(1):90.

7. Tang LL, Chen WQ, Xue WQ, et al. Global trends in incidence and mortality of nasopharyngeal carcinoma. Cancer Lett 2016;374(1):22–30.

8. Chan AT, Grégoire V, Lefebvre JL, et al. Nasopharyngeal cancer: EHNS-ESMO-ESTRO Clinical Practice Guidelines for diagnosis, treatment and follow-up. Ann Oncol 2012;23(Suppl 7):vii83–5.

9. Lee AW, Ma BB, Ng WT, et al. Management of nasopharyngeal carcinoma: current practice and future perspective. J Clin Oncol 2015;33(29):3356–64.

10. Mukherji SK, Castillo M. Normal cross-sectional anatomy of the nasopharynx, oropharynx, and oral cavity. Neuroimaging Clin North Am 1998;8(1): 211–8.

11. Chong VF, Ong CK. Nasopharyngeal carcinoma. Eur J Radiol 2008;66(3):437–47.

12. Pan WR, Suami H, Corlett RJ, et al. Lymphatic drainage of the nasal fossae and nasopharynx: preliminary anatomical and radiological study with clinical implications. Head Neck 2009;31(1):52–7.

13. Mukherji SK, Armao D, Joshi VM. Cervical nodal metastases in squamous cell carcinoma of the head and neck: what to expect. Head Neck 2001;23(11): 995–1005.

14. Emami B, Sethi A, Petruzzelli GJ. Influence of MRI on target volume delineation and IMRT planning in nasopharyngeal carcinoma. Int J Radiat Oncol Biol Phys 2003;57(2):481–8.

15. Chu HR, Kim JH, Yoon DY, et al. Additional diagnostic value of (18)F-FDG PET-CT in detecting retropharyngeal nodal metastases. Otolaryngol Head Neck Surg 2009;141(5):633–8.

16. Coskun HH, Ferlito A, Medina JE, et al. Retropharyngeal lymph node metastases in head and neck malignancies. Head Neck 2011;33(10):1520–9.

17. Metser U, Miller E, Lerman H, et al. Benign nonphysiologic lesions with increased 18F-FDG uptake on PET/CT: characterization and incidence. AJR Am J Roentgenol 2007;189(5):1203–10.

18. Kattan MW, Hess KR, Amin MB, et al. American Joint Committee on Cancer acceptance criteria for inclusion of risk models for individualized prognosis in the practice of precision medicine. CA Cancer J Clin 2016;66(5):370–4.

19. Amin MB, Greene FL, Edge SB, et al. The Eighth Edition AJCC Cancer Staging Manual: continuing to build a bridge from a population-based to a more "personalized" approach to cancer staging. CA Cancer J Clin 2017;67(2):93–9.

20. Chen WS, Li JJ, Hong L, et al. Comparison of MRI, CT and 18F-FDG PET/CT in the diagnosis of local and metastatic of nasopharyngeal carcinomas: an updated meta analysis of clinical studies. Am J Transl Res 2016;8(11):4532–47.

21. Liao X-B, Mao Y-P, Liu L-Z, et al. How does magnetic resonance imaging Influence staging according to AJCC staging system for nasopharyngeal carcinoma compared with computed tomography? Int J Radiat Oncol Biol Phys 2008;72(5):1368–77.

22. Ng SH, Chan SC, Yen TC, et al. Staging of untreated nasopharyngeal carcinoma with PET/CT: comparison with conventional imaging work-up. Eur J Nucl Med Mol Imaging 2009;36(1):12–22.

23. Lai V, Li X, Lee VHF, et al. Nasopharyngeal carcinoma: comparison of diffusion and perfusion characteristics between different tumour stages using intravoxel incoherent motion MR imaging. Eur Radiol 2014;24(1):176–83.

24. Mao J, Shen J, Yang Q, et al. Intravoxel incoherent motion MRI in differentiation between recurrent carcinoma and postchemoradiation fibrosis of the skull base in patients with nasopharyngeal carcinoma. J Magn Reson Imaging 2016;44(6):1556–64.

25. Chang K-P, Tsang N-M, Liao C-T, et al. Prognostic significance of ^{18}F-FDG PET parameters and plasma Epstein-barr virus DNA load in patients with nasopharyngeal carcinoma. J Nucl Med 2012; 53(1):21–8.

26. Peng H, Chen L, Tang LL, et al. Significant value of (18)F-FDG-PET/CT in diagnosing small cervical lymph node metastases in patients with nasopharyngeal carcinoma treated with intensity-modulated radiotherapy. Chin J Cancer 2017;36(1):95.

27. Shen G, Xiao W, Han F, et al. Advantage of PET/CT in target delineation of MRI-negative cervical lymph nodes in intensity-modulated radiation therapy planning for nasopharyngeal carcinoma. J Cancer 2017; 8(19):4117–23.

28. Aktan M, Kanyilmaz G, Yavuz BB, et al. Prognostic value of pre-treatment 18F-FDG PET uptake for nasopharyngeal carcinoma. Radiol Med 2017.

29. Lee SJ, Kay CS, Kim YS, et al. Prognostic value of nodal SUVmax of 18F-FDG PET/CT in nasopharyngeal carcinoma treated with intensity-modulated radiotherapy. Radiat Oncol J 2017;35(4):306–16.

30. King AD, Ma BB, Yau YY, et al. The impact of 18F-FDG PET/CT on assessment of nasopharyngeal carcinoma at diagnosis. Br J Radiol 2008;81(964): 291–8.

31. Chan SC, Yeh CH, Yen TC, et al. Clinical utility of simultaneous whole-body (18)F-FDG PET/MRI as a single-step imaging modality in the staging of primary nasopharyngeal carcinoma. Eur J Nucl Med Mol Imaging 2018;45(8):1297–308.

32. Chua MLK, Ong SC, Wee JTS, et al. Comparison of 4 modalities for distant metastasis staging in endemic nasopharyngeal carcinoma. Head Neck 2009;31(3):346–54.

33. Lim T, Chua M, Chia G, et al. Comparison of MRI, CT and 18F-FDG-PET/CT for the detection of intracranial disease extension in nasopharyngeal carcinoma. J Head Neck Oncol 2012;4(2):49.

34. Liu F, Xi XP, Wang H, et al. PET/CT-guided dose-painting versus CT-based intensity modulated radiation therapy in locoregional advanced nasopharyngeal carcinoma. Radiat Oncol 2017;12(1):15.

35. Wu VW, Leung WS, Wong KL, et al. The impact of positron emission tomography on primary tumour delineation and dosimetric outcome in intensity modulated radiotherapy of early T-stage nasopharyngeal carcinoma. Radiat Oncol 2016;11(1):109.

36. Chen YK, Su CT, Ding HJ, et al. Clinical usefulness of fused PET/CT compared with PET alone or CT alone in nasopharyngeal carcinoma patients. Anticancer Res 2006;26(2b):1471–7.

37. Xie P, Yue JB, Fu Z, et al. Prognostic value of 18F-FDG PET/CT before and after radiotherapy for locally advanced nasopharyngeal carcinoma. Ann Oncol 2010;21(5):1078–82.

38. Liu T, Xu W, Yan WL, et al. MRI for diagnosis of local residual or recurrent nasopharyngeal carcinoma, which one is the best? A systematic review. Radiother Oncol 2007;85(3):327–35.

39. Wei J, Pei S, Zhu X. Comparison of (18)F-FDG PET/CT, MRI and SPECT in the diagnosis of local residual/recurrent nasopharyngeal carcinoma: a meta-analysis. Oral Oncol 2016;52:11–7.

40. Porceddu SV, Jarmolowski E, Hicks RJ, et al. Utility of positron emission tomography for the detection of disease in residual neck nodes after (chemo) radiotherapy in head and neck cancer. Head Neck 2005;27(3):175–81.

41. Castaldi P, Leccisotti L, Bussu F, et al. Role of (18)F-FDG PET-CT in head and neck squamous cell carcinoma. Acta Otorhinolaryngol Ital 2013;33(1):1–8.

42. Andrade RS, Heron DE, Degirmenci B, et al. Post-treatment assessment of response using FDG-PET/CT for patients treated with definitive radiation therapy for head and neck cancers. Int J Radiat Oncol Biol Phys 2006;65(5):1315–22.

43. Liu S-H, Chang JT, Ng S-H, et al. False positive fluorine-18 fluorodeoxy-D-glucose positron emission tomography finding caused by osteoradionecrosis in a nasopharyngeal carcinoma patient. Br J Radiol 2004;77(915):257–60.

44. Bisdas S, Chambron Pinho N, Smolarz A, et al. Bisphosphonate-induced osteonecrosis of the jaws: CT and MRI spectrum of findings in 32 patients. Clin Radiol 2008;63(1):71–7.

45. King AD, Griffith JF, Abrigo JM, et al. Osteoradionecrosis of the upper cervical spine: MR imaging following radiotherapy for nasopharyngeal carcinoma. Eur J Radiol 2010;73(3):629–35.

46. Kim EE, Chung SK, Haynie TP, et al. Differentiation of residual or recurrent tumors from post-treatment changes with F-18 FDG PET. Radiographics 1992; 12(2):269–79.

47. Ricci PE, Karis JP, Heiserman JE, et al. Differentiating recurrent tumor from radiation necrosis: time for re-evaluation of positron emission tomography? AJNR Am J Neuroradiol 1998;19(3):407–13.

48. Purohit BS, Ailianou A, Dulguerov N, et al. FDG-PET/CT pitfalls in oncological head and neck imaging. Insights Imaging 2014;5(5):585–602.

49. Kostakoglu L, Hardoff R, Mirtcheva R, et al. PET-CT fusion imaging in differentiating physiologic from pathologic FDG uptake. Radiographics 2004;24(5): 1411–31.

50. Bhargava P, Rahman S, Wendt J. Atlas of confounding factors in head and neck PET/CT imaging. Clin Nucl Med 2011;36(5):e20–9.

51. Bi WL, Hosny A, Schabath MB, et al. Artificial intelligence in cancer imaging: clinical challenges and applications. CA Cancer J Clin 2019;69(2):127–57.

52. Aerts HJ. The potential of radiomic-based phenotyping in precision medicine: a review. JAMA Oncol 2016;2(12):1636–42.

53. Du D, Feng H, Lv W, et al. Machine learning methods for optimal radiomics-based differentiation between recurrence and inflammation: application to nasopharyngeal carcinoma post-therapy PET/CT images. Mol Imaging Biol 2020;22(3):730–8.

54. Lv W, Yuan Q, Wang Q, et al. Robustness versus disease differentiation when varying parameter settings in radiomics features: application to nasopharyngeal PET/CT. Eur Radiol 2018;28(8):3245–54.

55. Lv W, Yuan Q, Wang Q, et al. Radiomics analysis of PET and CT components of PET/CT imaging Integrated with clinical parameters: application to prognosis for nasopharyngeal carcinoma. Mol Imaging Biol 2019;21(5):954–64.

56. Xie C, Du R, Ho JW, et al. Effect of machine learning re-sampling techniques for imbalanced datasets in (18)F-FDG PET-based radiomics model on prognostication performance in cohorts of head and neck cancer patients. Eur J Nucl Med Mol Imaging 2020;47(12):2826–35.

57. Peng L, Hong X, Yuan Q, et al. Prediction of local recurrence and distant metastasis using radiomics

analysis of pretreatment nasopharyngeal [18F]FDG PET/CT images. Ann Nucl Med 2021.

58. Xu H, Lv W, Feng H, et al. Subregional radiomics analysis of PET/CT imaging with intratumor partitioning: application to prognosis for nasopharyngeal carcinoma. Mol Imaging Biol 2020;22(5):1414–26.

59. Peng H, Dong D, Fang MJ, et al. Prognostic value of deep learning PET/CT-based radiomics: potential role for future individual induction chemotherapy in advanced nasopharyngeal carcinoma. Clin Cancer Res 2019;25(14):4271–9.

60. Zhao L, Lu Z, Jiang J, et al. Automatic nasopharyngeal carcinoma segmentation using fully convolutional networks with auxiliary paths on dual-modality PET-CT images. J Digit Imaging 2019; 32(3):462–70.

PET/CT
Radiation Therapy Planning in Head and Neck Cancer

Salman Eraj, MD, David J. Sher, MD, MPH*

KEYWORDS

• PET/CT • Radiation planning • Adaptive radiotherapy

KEY POINTS

• Modern radiotherapy offers highly conformal treatment that requires accurate delineation of primary and nodal targets to achieve optimal cancer control with reduced toxicity.
• FDG-PET/CT has an integral role in guiding target delineation in radiotherapy planning for most head and neck cancers.
• Efforts are underway investigating the use of pre- and mid-treatment PET/CT to guide radiation dose and volume escalation/de-escalation approaches.

INTRODUCTION

The combination of functional imaging with fluorine-18-fluorodeoxyglucose (FDG) positron emission tomography (PET) and anatomic imaging with computed tomography (CT) has become an indispensable tool in the assessment of head and neck cancers. Other articles in this issue describe the use of PET/CT in specific sites for staging, assessment of therapy response, and for posttherapy follow-up. This article reviews the use of PET/CT in radiotherapy planning. First, the evolution of radiotherapy and the need for improved target definition beyond that provided by anatomic imaging is described. The current role of PET in standard target definition, dose, and volume modification for escalation/de-escalation, and adaptive radiotherapy follows. Lastly, there is a brief overview of the use of alternative PET tracers and biologically guided radiation therapy.

MODERN RADIOTHERAPY

Over the past several decades, head and neck radiotherapy have experienced significant technical improvements through the use of 3D conformal radiotherapy (3D-CRT), intensity-modulated radiotherapy (IMRT), image-guided radiotherapy (IGRT), and proton therapy. In 3D-CRT, treatment planning is performed by choosing radiation beam directions that would best target the tumor and spare normal structures, and shaping each beam with a multileaf collimator (MLC) to fit the profile of the target with margin. IMRT is an evolution of 3D-CRT whereby the intensity of the radiation beams is modulated by the MLC segments with either multiple, cross-firing, static beams or with arc therapy, which delivers radiation while the arm of the linear accelerator is in motion. IMRT has been compared with 3D-CRT in multiple trials and has been shown to offer high tumor control rates with reduced toxicity, significantly lowering the rates of xerostomia from reduced dose to the salivary glands, and it is considered the standard-of-care in the modern management of head and neck cancer radiotherapy.[1–3] Proton therapy uses protons for delivery of radiation dose as opposed to standard photon-based treatments, leveraging the fact that protons deposit most of their energy at the end of their paths in the target, with minimal exit dose to decrease dose to organs at risk (OARs).

Department of Radiation Oncology, University of Texas Southwestern Medical Center, 2280 Inwood Drive, Dallas, TX 75390, USA
* Corresponding author.
E-mail address: David.sher@utsouthwestern.edu

PET Clin 17 (2022) 297–305
https://doi.org/10.1016/j.cpet.2021.12.007

These highly conformal therapies have dramatically amplified the need for accurate target delineation.

RADIOTHERAPY TREATMENT PLANNING

To plan radiotherapy, a CT scan is performed in the treatment position in a process called a simulation. The CT provides anatomic and electron density information that is critical for treatment planning. In radiotherapy for head and neck cancer, immobilization typically involves the creation of a thermoplastic mask that will be used for all subsequent treatments. Following simulation, the volumes of interest must be delineated or "contoured" on the acquired images. The International Commission on Radiation Units and Measurements (ICRU) published a widely accepted nomenclature that defined volumes of interest in radiotherapy, including the gross tumor volume (GTV), clinical target volume (CTV), and planning target volume (PTV).[4,5] The GTV is the volume that contains the gross tumor defined by clinical examination and radiographic studies of the primary site and involved lymph nodes (LN). The CTV is the volume containing the GTV and any suspected local or regional microscopic disease and is important because this volume must be adequately treated to achieve cure. Within head and neck cancer radiotherapy, the CTV includes the volume around the GTVs, often using a 5 to 10 mm 3D expansion, but also the at-risk nodal groups that may harbor microscopic disease. The PTV is the volume created with an additional margin around the GTV and CTV (typically 3–5 mm) to account for daily uncertainties in treatment, such as organ/patient motion and setup errors (**Fig. 1**). In principle, coverage of the PTV with the prescription dose ensures sufficient delivery of this dose to the CTV.

Given the desire to deliver conformal treatments with sharp dose gradients to spare adjacent organs-at-risk (OARs, or normal tissue), accurate target delineation and careful specification of desired dose distributions are crucial. In head and neck cancer radiotherapy, the GTV, including the primary tumor and involved LNs, are at the highest dose level. There are often multiple CTVs that receive varying lower doses to account for microscopic disease. The American Joint Committee of Cancer Staging and a working group with representation from major relevant cooperative groups in radiation oncology have classified lymph nodes groups in the head and neck and given recommendations for the delineation of neck node levels on axial CT sections.[6,7] Highly conformal treatments can lead to unrecognized microscopic disease not being included in the necessary volume, resulting in locoregional failures. Alternatively, overly generous target volumes can result in additional dose to OARs that may lead to increased toxicities.

FDG-POSITRON EMISSION TOMOGRAPHY/COMPUTED TOMOGRAPHY IN PRIMARY TUMOR DELINEATION

The incorporation of PET/CT in radiotherapy treatment planning typically requires fusion of the PET portion of the examination to the CT being used for simulation. As PET/CT is often obtained in the workup of patients who will go on to receive radiotherapy, one common approach consists of image registration of the diagnostic PET/CT to the subsequent simulation CT. Accuracy of image registration is limited in this approach by the differences in patient positioning, weight changes, and tumor growth/response between the scans. Although a variety of rigid and deformable registration solutions have been developed to address this, inaccuracies remain and more ideal approaches include the acquisition of PET/CT in the simulation position with immobilization, either following CT simulation or with the use of a PET/CT simulator.[8]

Numerous studies have investigated the value of PET/CT in the primary target delineation of the GTV, but the fundamental question is how the PET/CT data are used to accurately define the gross disease. Visual interpretation is the most commonly used method, but it is sensitive to window-level settings and is operator-dependent. More objective methods include, but are not limited to, isocontouring based on a specific absolute SUV, a fixed relative threshold of the SUVmax, or a threshold that is adaptive to the signal-to-noise ratio. Specifically, one of the most used automatic segmentation methods is to use an SUV threshold, between 2 and 3 (absolute value) or 40% to 50% (relative value of SUVmax). In a study of 29 patients with stage II–IV HNSCC, comparison of GTVs delineated on CT, MR imaging, and PET/CT were compared and correlated with pathologic surgical specimens.[9] For PET, 10 oropharyngeal GTVs were delineated using a segmentation algorithm based on the measured signal-to-noise ratio and were generally found to be smaller than and not totally encompassed by those delineated on CT ($P = .02$) or MR imaging ($P = .10$); there were similar results in 19 patients with laryngeal and hypopharyngeal tumors.[10] In a review of the 9 patients who underwent laryngectomy, the average surgical tumor volume was significantly smaller than those delineated radiographically, with PET/CT being the most accurate, although all modalities underestimated

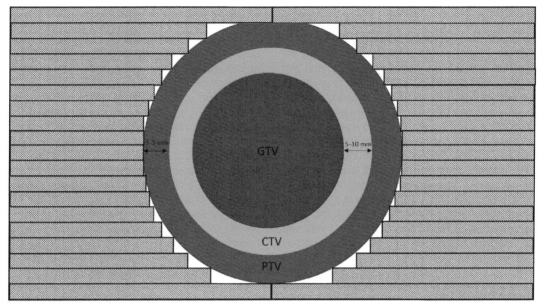

Fig. 1. Schematic representation of gross tumor volume (GTV), clinical target volume (CTV), planning target volume (PTV) with conformal multi-leaf collimation.

superficial tumor extension. On average, 10%, 9%, and 13% of the GTVs contoured from CT, MR imaging, and PET/CT, respectively, were delineated only from the macroscopic surgical specimen. Visual interpretation and automatic segmentation of PET/CT have been studied in other series and demonstrated similar results, with generally smaller primary tumor GTV using PET/CT compared with other imaging modalities.[11–15]

Indeed, retrospective studies have suggested that FDG-PET/CT can help identify volumes at risk for treatment failure and thus ensure adequate coverage in planning. For instance, a study by Mohamed and colleagues analyzed 47 patients with local/regional recurrence following definitive IMRT with pretreatment PET/CT available to identify the radio-resistant subvolumes.[16] The recurrent GTVs were delineated, and the nidus volume (NV) of recurrence (center of mass plus 4 mm margin) was identified. Forty-two (89.4%) patients had a central high dose failure whereby 95% of the recurrent GTV received ≥95% of the corresponding target volume prescription dose. Forty-eight percent of these failures were at the primary site and the remainder was in a nodal basin, with a mean prior dose to recurrent GTVs of 71 Gy. The authors considered whether PET/CT could identify the regions at highest risk for failure and thus be boosted with additional radiotherapy. Multiple boost volumes using thresholds of 30% to 70% of the preradiotherapy SUVmax and variable margins were analyzed for coverage of the nidus volume. A boost volume consisting of 50% of

SUVmax plus a 10 mm margin was identified as the optimal subvolume with high nidus volume coverage (92.3%), low average relative volume to the original high-dose CTV (41%), and the least average percent voxels outside original high-dose CTV (19%). Whether or not dose escalation would be successful is a separate clinical question (to be discussed later), but these data showing that pretreatment PET/CT can identify volumes at highest risk for failure emphasize the impact of the imaging study on routine target delineation.

FDG-POSITRON EMISSION TOMOGRAPHY/COMPUTED TOMOGRAPHY IN LYMPH NODE DELINEATION

The utility of PET/CT to define malignant adenopathy is well-established and is regularly used in clinical practice to identify the lymph node GTV, recognizing that the operating characteristics are still not sufficient to be the sole modality. For example, the American College of Radiology Imaging Network (ACRIN) 6685 trial was a multi-center prospective study of PET/CT in patients presenting with cT2-T4N0 HNSCC.[17] All patients underwent neck dissection of the side ipsilateral to the primary with blinded PET/CT before surgery. By visual assessment, the NPV specific to the cN0 sides was 0.87 (95% confidence interval (CI): 0.80–0.93). With the use of prespecified cutoffs of 2.5 and 3.5 SUVmax, the NPVs specific to the nodal basins were 0.940 (95% CI: 0.928–0.952) and 0.937 (95% CI: 0.925–0.949), respectively. The optimal cutoff SUVmax value was determined to be 1.8, with an NPV of 0.942 (95% CI: 0.930–0.953), but specificity naturally suffered. The PET/CT-informed surgical treatment plan was changed in 51 of 237 participants (22%) compared with the PET/CT-blinded surgical plan. While this study was primarily geared toward primary surgical therapy, these diagnostic rules can inform radiation oncologists' target design, as the decision can be difficult on whether an identified lymph node is suspicious enough to receive a higher dose.

The optimal analysis method by which a radiation oncologist should define a lymph node as positive and therefore, GTV is unclear. A study by Schinagl demonstrated that both CT and visually interpreted PET/CT-based nodal volumes showed good correlation with subsequent pathologic specimens, but interestingly, visual interpretation was as accurate as any segmentation algorithm.[18] On the other hand, a study by Sadick and colleagues evaluated the performance of PET/CT in 123 LNs in 33 patients using a threshold of SUVmax $\geq$3 to define LN positivity with postoperative histology serving as the gold standard.[19] Sensitivity and PPV were 100% and 93%, respectively, and specificity and NPV were 87% and 100%, respectively.

Ultimately, the goal of improved target delineation is improved outcomes, and thus the results from a large, retrospective study from the Netherlands that evaluated the impact of FDG-PET/CT based nodal target volume delineation on survival are compelling.[20] Forty-six percent of the included 693 patients had PET guided nodal volumes using visual analysis with a median follow-up of 31 months. Patients whose nodal volumes were guided by PET experienced improved disease control in the elective CTV (HR: 0.33, P = .026), overall regional control (HR: 0.62, P = .027), and overall survival (HR: 0.71, P = .033) compared with patient with CT based volumes.

FDG-POSITRON EMISSION TOMOGRAPHY/COMPUTED TOMOGRAPHY-GUIDED DOSE MODIFICATION AND RESPONSE-ADAPTED ADAPTIVE RADIOTHERAPY

Despite the aforementioned improvements in imaging and target delineation afforded by the use of PET/CT, locoregional recurrence remains a common mode of treatment failure in patients with HNSCC, particularly in those with HPV-negative disease or smoking history.[21–24] One strategy that has been explored to address these recurrences is dose escalation, in which targets at highest risk for recurrence (ie, subvolumes) are boosted to a higher radiation dose. FDG-PET/CT

has been used to guide subvolume definition in some studies of dose escalation, but there is significant heterogeneity within and between these studies in terms of radiation dosing, systemic therapy, disease characteristics, and outcome reporting, constraining useful comparisons.[25–31]

Radiation oncologists in Belgium have pioneered PET-guided dose escalation approaches with dose painting of subvolumes within the target. Their initial phase I study used "dose painting by contour" (DPBC), whereby the dose was homogenously escalated inside the PET defined contour within the GTV.[32] The PET defined contour was the result of automatic segmentation of the PET images, based on the signal-to-noise ratio. Patients received an upfront simultaneous integrated boost with 2 dose levels of 25 Gy and 30 Gy in 10 fractions followed by 22 fractions of 2.16 Gy, leading to a total escalated dose equivalent to 75 Gy and 81 Gy in 2 Gy fractions, respectively, clearly higher than the accepted standard of 70 Gy. There were 2 cases of dose-limiting toxicity (out of 23 patients) at the 25 Gy dose level, and one treatment-related death (out of 18) at the 30 Gy level, but overall the treatment was well tolerated and the maximum tolerated dose was not reached. Despite the escalated dose, in 4 of 9 patients who recurred, the site of relapse was directly in the boosted region.

PET/CT obtained during a course of radiotherapy, or interim PET, has demonstrated that PET-based target volumes often shrink during treatment.[33] This observation has led to the study of response-adapted adaptive radiotherapy, whereby cumulative tumor or subvolume dose is increased or decreased based on metabolic response. The same group from Belgium has investigated this approach with adaptive "dose painting by number" (A-DPBN), whereby rather than using PET to create a discrete boost volume to receive a homogenous dose, the range of PET voxel intensities is used to create heterogeneous dose distributions within the target, escalating dose to the most metabolically active and theoretically radioresistant portions of the GTV. This group has conducted two phase I trials investigating this approach, adapting treatment using PET/CT obtained after either 8 fractions or after 8 and 18 fractions.[34–36] In the three-phase A-DPBN study, 2 dose prescription levels were tested: a median dose of 80.9 Gy to the high-dose CTV (dose level I) in 7 patients and a median dose of 85.9 Gy to the gross tumor volume (GTV) (dose level II) in 14 patients. The restaging PET/CT scans were performed during radiotherapy and thus the treatment volumes were changed twice over the course of treatment, reducing the volumes.

Treatment adaptation reduced the volumes of the GTV (41%, P = .01), high-dose CTV (18%, P = .01), high-dose PTV (14%, P = .02), and parotids (9%–12%, P < .05). There were no treatment breaks and no grade 4 acute toxicity was observed. A subsequent study compared 72 patients enrolled on the group's 3 dose escalation trials to 72 control patients matched on tumor site and T classification that received standard IMRT.[28] A total median dose to the dose-painted target was 70.2-85.9 Gy/30-32 fractions versus 69.1 Gy/32 fractions with conventional IMRT. Five-year local control rate in the dose-painted patients was 82.3% versus 73.6% in the matched controls (P = .36). There was no statistical difference in regional (P = .82) and distant control (P = .78), or 5-year overall (P = .50) and disease-specific (P = .72) survival rates. Acute grade $\geq$3 dysphagia was observed in 54%, 52%, and 30% of patients treated with DPBC, 2-phase A-DPBN, and 3-phase A-DPBN, respectively (P = .01), compared with 26% of patients treated with standard IMRT (P = .004, between all study and control patients). Significantly higher rates of late dysphagia were also seen in the study patients (P = .005). These data suggest that while PET/CT-based escalation may be feasible, it is an open question whether this paradigm will prove to be beneficial.

Indeed, the completed, but not yet published, ARTFORCE randomized phase III study compares standard radiotherapy of 70 Gy in 35 fractions to a dosing regimen in which a subvolume of the primary tumor receives a higher dose based on 50% SUVmax in the primary tumor.[37] The PET guided GTV receives up to 84 Gy (and a mean around 77 Gy), with the primary outside of the PET guided GTV meant to receive a mean dose of 67 Gy.[38] The study is powered for locoregional control and to show a 15% improvement with dose escalation. The results of this study should give the clearest evidence to date on the outcomes associated with PET-guided dose escalation.

FDG-POSITRON EMISSION TOMOGRAPHY/COMPUTED TOMOGRAPHY-GUIDED DOSE DE-ESCALATION

The basic radiotherapy treatment paradigm for HNSCC consists of a radical dose of 66 to 70 Gy to the gross primary and nodal disease with routine prophylactic (or "elective") treatment of the bilateral neck to a dose of 56 to 63 Gy. In contrast to cancers that are typically caused by smoking-related behavior, the feasibility of treatment de-escalation seems particularly feasible with favorable HPV-positive oropharynx cancer,

with phase II studies showing that reduced-dose to only 54 to 60 Gy may lead to durable tumor control.[39–41] On the other hand, there is some concern that unselected dose de-escalation may cause an unacceptably high locoregional failure rate. The University of Michigan is performing a phase II study using interim FDG-PET/CT to de-escalate the total dose to 54 Gy, but only among patients with a favorable response to interim PET/CT after several weeks of treatment.[42]

In addition, the overall volume of GTV matters as well, with smaller volumes naturally leading to lower doses to normal tissues, and PET/CT may have a benefit in defining this smaller volume. There is an actively recruiting phase II feasibility study, PET-based Adaptive Radiotherapy Clinical Trial (PEARL), investigating de-escalation in HPV positive and node-positive oropharynx cancer using interim PET/CT.[43–47] In this study, PET/CT will be used to guide initial planning, with an interim PET/CT after 2 weeks of chemoradiation used to redistribute dose in patients with early metabolic response and shrink the high-dose GTV. Thus, patients whose metabolic tumor volume shrinks over those first 2 weeks will experience a potentially meaningful reduction in the volume receiving the highest dose.

Another paradigm of treatment de-escalation involves reducing or even eliminating the dose to the elective neck. Although historically cervical lymph nodes are comprehensively treated to sterilize micrometastatic disease, the risk of solitary elective recurrences is on the order of 0% to 3% with the use of standard doses of $\geq$50 Gy.[48–53] A study by van den Bosch evaluated 1166 LNs and demonstrated that elective nodal recurrence always occurred in a previously visualized (presumed benign) LN, thus supporting the premise that at-risk LNs are visible at diagnosis.

A recently published phase II trial of radiotherapy dose and volume de-escalation ("INFIELD") from our institution leveraged FDG-PET/CT data to define lymph nodes as involved or suspicious and then treated the remaining elective neck dose to 40 Gy or eliminated it altogether, depending on the location of the station.[54] Involved nodes received 70 Gy and were defined by enlarged size ($\geq$1 cm short axis, 1.5 cm in level II), internal necrosis, or SUVmax greater than 3.0. "Suspicious" LNs were treated to 64 Gy and were defined by axial cross-sectional summed diameter $\geq$17 mm or SUVmax > internal jugular vein blood pool uptake (visual analysis, Hopkins criteria score 2). At a median follow-up of 24.7 months for surviving patients, there were no solitary elective nodal recurrences, showing the clinical benefit of the high negative predictive value of FDG-PET/CT. Our institution then completed a successor trial ("INRT-AIR") for which the elective neck dose was completely abandoned, targeting only nodes as involved or suspicious based on PET/CT, CT, and an artificial intelligence algorithm incorporating both imaging modalities.[55]

ALTERNATIVE TRACERS

In addition to the use of FDG as a PET tracer, there are other tracers that function as indicators of hypoxia, such as fluorine-18-fluoroazomycin-arabinoside (FAZA) and fluorine-18-fluoromisonidazole (FMISO), that are being investigated to guide the modification of treatment intensity.[56,57] A recent example is the 30 ROC trial, in which pre- and intratreatment FMISO-PET/CT from Memorial Sloan-Kettering Cancer Center were used to assess tumor hypoxia in 19 patients with HPV-positive oropharyngeal cancer whose primary tumor was treated with surgery.[58] If there were no hypoxic regions seen by the interim FMISO-PET/CT, the total dose to the nodes was stopped at only 30 Gy. In total, 15 patients received this de-escalated treatment, with surprisingly favorable outcomes of 11 pathologic complete responses and 2-year locoregional control of 94.4% (95% CI: 84.4%–100%) and overall survival of 94.7% (95% CI: 85.2%–100%). This somewhat remarkable result has prompted subsequent trials of FMISO-based treatment at this institution, ultimately including the primary disease as a candidate for this dramatic dose de-escalation.

POSITRON EMISSION TOMOGRAPHY/ COMPUTED TOMOGRAPHY -GUIDED RADIOTHERAPY

In the most direct application of PET/CT to radiotherapy, a new type of linear accelerator has been developed (Reflexion, Reflexion Medical) that uses the PET/CT signal to guide treatment, a concept termed Biologically guided Radiation Therapy (BgRT). Before entering the machine for each fraction, patients are given a dose of FDG. The basic premise of this technology is that the machine can deliver therapeutic radiation in a direct anatomic response to detecting an emitted positron from the patient, thus allowing extremely precise and compact dose delivery. The PET signal effectively serves as a biological fiducial, targeting the treatment and reducing the required safety margins (ie, PTV), thus lowering the dose to normal tissues. For example, the difference in PTV volume may be more than 50% smaller (40.7%–55.9%) in lung stereotactic applications.[59] In principle, the fusing of a therapeutic and

diagnostic machine may also lead to on-board PET/CT-based adaptive radiotherapy using a variety of exciting tracers.

SUMMARY

Just as FDG-PET/CT has become a standard staging and restaging modality in HNSCC, so too has it become an indispensable part of radiotherapy planning. The study is not only a routinely used tool in primary and nodal target delineation but also has an emerging role in guiding adaptive escalation and de-escalation efforts. Continued collaboration between radiation oncologists and nuclear medicine physicians is essential to identify novel imaging and treatment paradigms that can optimize the therapeutic ratio.

CLINICS CARE POINTS

- FDG-PET/CT imaging should be used to facilitate contouring for patients treated with definitive head and neck radiotherapy.

- It is preferable to perform the PET-/CT in the treatment position with immobilization, but if this arrangement is not possible, pay particular attention to the quality of the image fusion.

- Dose escalation or de-escalation as a function of FDG-PET/CT imaging may be feasible in the future, but the current evidence is still insufficient to support this approach.

DISCLOSURE

The authors have nothing to disclose.

REFERENCES

1. Nutting CM, Morden JP, Harrington KJ, et al. Parotid-sparing intensity modulated versus conventional radiotherapy in head and neck cancer (PARSPORT): a phase 3 multicentre randomised controlled trial. Lancet Oncol 2011;12(2):127–36.

2. Eisbruch A, Harris J, Garden AS, et al. Multi-institutional trial of accelerated hypofractionated intensity-modulated radiation therapy for early-stage oropharyngeal cancer (RTOG 00-22). Int J Radiat Oncol Biol Phys 2010;76(5):1333–8.

3. Tao Y, Auperin A, Blanchard P, et al. Concurrent cisplatin and dose escalation with intensity-modulated radiotherapy (IMRT) versus conventional radiotherapy for locally advanced head and neck

squamous cell carcinomas (HNSCC): GORTEC 2004-01 randomized phase III trial. Radiother Oncol 2020;150:18–25.

4. Landberg T, Chavaudra J, Dobbs J, et al. Report 50. J Int Comm Radiat Units Meas 1993;os26(1):NP. https://doi.org/10.1093/jicru/os26.1. Report50.

5. Landberg T, Chavaudra J, Dobbs J, et al. Report 62. J Int Comm Radiat Units Meas 1999;os32(1):NP. https://doi.org/10.1093/jicru/os32.1. Report62.

6. Edge Stephen B, Amin Mahul B, Meyer Laura R, et al. American Joint Committee on cancer. AJCC cancer staging Manual. 8th edition. Springer; 2017. https://doi.org/10.3322/caac.21388.

7. Grégoire V, Ang K, Budach W, et al. Delineation of the neck node levels for head and neck tumors: a 2013 update. DAHANCA, EORTC, HKNPCSG, NCIC CTG, NCRI, RTOG, TROG consensus guidelines. Radiother Oncol 2014;110(1):172–81.

8. Hwang AB, Bacharach SL, Yom SS, et al. Can positron emission tomography (PET) or PET/computed tomography (CT) acquired in a Nontreatment position Be accurately registered to a head-and-neck radiotherapy planning CT? Int J Radiat Oncol Biol Phys 2009;73(2):578–84.

9. Daisne JF, Duprez T, Weynand B, et al. Tumor volume in pharyngolaryngeal squamous cell carcinoma: comparison at CT, MR imaging, and FDG PET and validation with surgical specimen. Radiology 2004;233(1):93–100.

10. Daisne JF, Sibomana M, Bol A, et al. Tri-dimensional automatic segmentation of PET volumes based on measured source-to-background ratios: influence of reconstruction algorithms. Radiother Oncol 2003;69(3):247–50.

11. Geets X, Daisne JF, Tomsej M, et al. Impact of the type of imaging modality on target volumes delineation and dose distribution in pharyngo-laryngeal squamous cell carcinoma: comparison between pre- and per-treatment studies. Radiother Oncol 2006;78(3):291–7.

12. Guido A, Fuccio L, Rombi B, et al. Combined 18F-FDG-PET/CT Imaging in radiotherapy target delineation for head-and-neck cancer. Int J Radiat Oncol Biol Phys 2009;73(3):759–63.

13. Heron DE, Andrade RS, Flickinger J, et al. Hybrid PET-CT simulation for radiation treatment planning in head-and-neck cancers: a brief technical report. Int J Radiat Oncol Biol Phys 2004;60(5):1419–24.

14. Paulino AC, Koshy M, Howell R, et al. Comparison of CT- and FDG-PET-defined gross tumor volume in intensity-modulated radiotherapy for head-and-neck cancer. Int J Radiat Oncol Biol Phys 2005; 61(5):1385–92.

15. Caldas-Magalhaes J, Kasperts N, Kooij N, et al. Validation of imaging with pathology in laryngeal cancer: accuracy of the registration methodology. Int J Radiat Oncol Biol Phys 2012;82(2):289–98.

16. Mohamed ASR, Cardenas CE, Garden AS, et al. Patterns-of-failure guided biological target volume definition for head and neck cancer patients: FDG-PET and dosimetric analysis of dose escalation candidate subregions. Radiother Oncol 2017;124(2): 248–55.

17. Lowe VJ, Duan F, Subramaniam RM, et al. Multicenter trial of [18F]fluorodeoxyglucose positron emission tomography/computed tomography staging of head and neck cancer and negative predictive value and surgical impact in the n0 neck: results from acrin 6685. J Clin Oncol 2019;37(20):1704–12.

18. Schinagl DAX, Span PN, Van Den Hoogen FJA, et al. Pathology-based validation of FDG PET segmentation tools for volume assessment of lymph node metastases from head and neck cancer. Eur J Nucl Med Mol Imaging 2013;40(12):1828–35.

19. Sadick M, Weiss C, Piniol R, et al. 18F-fluorodeoxyglucose uptake level-based lymph node staging in oropharyngeal squamous cell cancer role of molecular marker expression on diagnostic outcome. Oncol Res Treat 2015;38(1–2):16–22.

20. van den Bosch S, Doornaert PAH, Dijkema T, et al. 18F-FDG-PET/CT-based treatment planning for definitive (chemo)radiotherapy in patients with head and neck squamous cell carcinoma improves regional control and survival. Radiother Oncol 2020;142:107–14.

21. Chao KSC, Ozyigit G, Tran BN, et al. Patterns of failure in patients receiving definitive and postoperative IMRT for head-and-neck cancer. Int J Radiat Oncol Biol Phys 2003;55(2):312–21.

22. Leeman JE, gao Li J, Pei X, et al. Patterns of treatment failure and postrecurrence outcomes among patients with locally advanced head and neck squamous cell carcinoma after chemoradiotherapy using modern radiation techniques. JAMA Oncol 2017; 3(11):1487–94.

23. Solomon CG, Grotta JC. Carotid stenosis. N Engl J Med 2013;369(12):1143–50.

24. Ang KK, Harris J, Wheeler R, et al. Human papillomavirus and survival of patients with oropharyngeal cancer. N Engl J Med 2010;363(1):24–35.

25. Atwell D, Elks J, Cahill K, et al. A review of modern radiation therapy dose escalation in locally advanced head and neck cancer. Clin Oncol 2020; 32(5):330–41.

26. Studer G, Peponi E, Kloeck S, et al. Surviving hypopharynx-larynx carcinoma in the era of IMRT. Int J Radiat Oncol Biol Phys 2010;77(5): 1391–6.

27. Welz S, Mönnich D, Pfannenberg C, et al. Prognostic value of dynamic hypoxia PET in head and neck cancer: results from a planned interim analysis of a randomized phase II hypoxia-image guided dose escalation trial. Radiother Oncol 2017;124(3): 526–32.

28. Berwouts D, Madani I, Duprez F, et al. Long-term outcome of 18F-fluorodeoxyglucose-positron emission tomography-guided dose painting for head and neck cancer: matched case-control study. Head Neck 2017;39(11):2264–75.

29. Bakst RL, Lee N, Pfister DG, et al. Hypofractionated dose-painting intensity modulated radiation therapy with chemotherapy for nasopharyngeal carcinoma: a prospective trial. Int J Radiat Oncol Biol Phys 2011;80(1):148–53.

30. Liu F, Xi X ping, Wang H, et al. PET/CT-guided dose-painting versus CT-based intensity modulated radiation therapy in locoregional advanced nasopharyngeal carcinoma. Radiat Oncol 2017; 12(1):1–10.

31. Wang J, Zheng J, Tang T, et al. A randomized pilot trial comparing Position Emission Tomography (PET)-guided dose escalation radiotherapy to conventional radiotherapy in chemoradiotherapy treatment of locally advanced nasopharyngeal carcinoma. PLoS One 2015;10(4):1–11.

32. Madani I, Duthoy W, Derie C, et al. Positron emission tomography-guided, focal-dose escalation using intensity-modulated radiotherapy for head and neck cancer. Int J Radiat Oncol Biol Phys 2007; 68(1):126–35.

33. Castadot P, Geets X, Lee JA, et al. Assessment by a deformable registration method of the volumetric and positional changes of target volumes and organs at risk in pharyngo-laryngeal tumors treated with concomitant chemo-radiation. Radiother Oncol 2010;95(2):209–17.

34. Berwouts D, Olteanu LAM, Duprez F, et al. Three-phase adaptive dose-painting-by-numbers for head-and-neck cancer: initial results of the phase i clinical trial. Radiother Oncol 2013;107(3):310–6.

35. Duprez F, De Neve W, De Gersem W, et al. Adaptive dose painting by numbers for head-and-neck cancer. Int J Radiat Oncol Biol Phys 2011;80(4):1045–55.

36. Madani I, Duprez F, Boterberg T, et al. Maximum tolerated dose in a phase i trial on adaptive dose painting by numbers for head and neck cancer. Radiother Oncol 2011;101(3):351–5.

37. Adaptive Radiation Treatment for Head and Neck Cancer (ARTFORCE). ClinicalTrials.gov identifer: NCT01504815. 2020. Available at: https://clinicaltrials.gov/ct2/show/NCT01504815.

38. Heukelom J, Hamming O, Bartelink H, et al. Adaptive and innovative radiation treatment FOR improving cancer treatment outcomE (ARTFORCE); a randomized controlled phase II trial for individualized treatment of head and neck cancer. BMC Cancer 2013;13:1–8.

39. Chen AM, Felix C, Wang PC, et al. Reduced-dose radiotherapy for human papillomavirus-associated squamous-cell carcinoma of the oropharynx: a single-arm, phase 2 study. Lancet Oncol 2017; 18(6):803–11.

40. Chera BS, Amdur RJ, Green R, et al. Phase II trial of de-intensified chemoradiotherapy for human papillomavirus–associated oropharyngeal squamous cell carcinoma. J Clin Oncol 2019;37(29): 2661–9.

41. Yom SS, Torres-Saavedra P, Caudell JJ, et al. Reduced-dose radiation therapy for HPV-associated oropharyngeal carcinoma (NRG Oncology HN002). J Clin Oncol 2021;39(9):956–65.

42. Individualized adaptive de-escalated radiotherapy for HPV-related oropharynx cancer. ClinicalTrials.gov identifier: NCT03416153. 2021. Available at: https://clinicaltrials.gov/ct2/show/NCT03416153.

43. Min M, Lin P, Lee MT, et al. Prognostic role of metabolic parameters of 18F-FDG PET-CT scan performed during radiation therapy in locally advanced head and neck squamous cell carcinoma. Eur J Nucl Med Mol Imaging 2015;42(13): 1984–94.

44. Lin P, Min M, Lee M, et al. Prognostic utility of 18F-FDG PET-CT performed prior to and during primary radiotherapy for nasopharyngeal carcinoma: index node is a useful prognostic imaging biomarker site. Radiother Oncol 2016;120(1):87–91.

45. Min M, Lin P, Lee M, et al. 18F-FDG PET-CT performed before and during radiation therapy of head and neck squamous cell carcinoma: are they independent or complementary to each other? J Med Imaging Radiat Oncol 2016;60(3): 433–40.

46. Mowery YM, Vergalasova I, Rushing CN, et al. Early 18F-FDG-PET response during radiation therapy for HPV-related oropharyngeal cancer may predict disease recurrence. Int J Radiat Oncol Biol Phys 2020; 108(4):969–76.

47. Bussink J, van Herpen CML, Kaanders JHAM, et al. PET-CT for response assessment and treatment adaptation in head and neck cancer. Lancet Oncol 2010;11(7):661–9.

48. Sher DJ, Thotakura V, Balboni TA, et al. Treatment of oropharyngeal squamous cell carcinoma with IMRT: patterns of failure after concurrent chemoradiotherapy and sequential therapy. Ann Oncol 2012;23(9): 2391–8.

49. Dandekar V, Morgan T, Turian J, et al. Patterns-of-failure after helical tomotherapy-based chemoradiotherapy for head and neck cancer: implications for CTV margin, elective nodal dose and bilateral parotid sparing. Oral Oncol 2014;50(5):520–6.

50. Garden AS, Dong L, Morrison WH, et al. Patterns of disease recurrence following treatment of oropharyngeal cancer with intensity modulated radiation therapy. Int J Radiat Oncol Biol Phys 2013;85. https://doi.org/10.1016/j.ijrobp.2012.08.004.

51. Huang K, Xia P, Chuang C, et al. Intensity-modulated chemoradiation for treatment of stage III and IV oropharyngeal carcinoma: the University of California-San Francisco experience. Cancer 2008; 113(3):497–507.

52. Duprez F, Bonte K, De Neve W, et al. Regional relapse after intensity-modulated radiotherapy for head-and-neck cancer. Int J Radiat Oncol Biol Phys 2011;79(2):450–8.

53. Van Den Bosch S, Dijkema T, Verhoef LCG, et al. Patterns of recurrence in electively irradiated lymph node regions after definitive accelerated intensity modulated radiation therapy for head and neck squamous cell Carcinoma. Int J Radiat Oncol Biol Phys 2016;94(4):766–74.

54. Sher DJ, Pham NL, Shah JL, et al. Prospective phase 2 study of radiation therapy dose and volume de-escalation for elective neck treatment of oropharyngeal and laryngeal cancer. Int J Radiat Oncol Biol Phys 2021;109(4):932–40.

55. INRT-AIR: A prospective phase II study of involved nodal radiation therapy. ClnicalTrais.gov identifier: NCT03953976. 2020. Available at: https://www.clinicaltrials.gov/ct2/show/NCT03953976.

56. Servagi-Vernat S, Differding S, Sterpin E, et al. Hypoxia-guided adaptive radiation dose escalation in head and neck carcinoma: a planning study. Acta Oncol (Madr) 2015;54(7):1008–16.

57. Halmos GB, De Bruin LB, Langendijk JA, et al. Head and neck tumor hypoxia imaging by 18F-fluoroazomycin- arabinoside (18F-FAZA)-PET: a review. Clin Nucl Med 2014;39(1):44–8.

58. Riaz N, Sherman E, Pei X, et al. Precision radiotherapy: reduction in radiation for oropharyngeal cancer in the 30 ROC trial. J Natl Cancer Inst 2021;00. https://doi.org/10.1093/jnci/djaa184.

59. Olcott P, Shirvani SM, Tian S, et al. Simultaneous integrated boost of lung tumors in the stereotactic ablative setting using BgRT tracked delivery. Int J Radiat Oncol 2020;108(3):e306.

2-Deoxy-2-[^{18}F] Fluoro-D-Glucose PET/Computed Tomography

Therapy Response Assessment in Head and Neck Cancer

Sara Sheikhbahaei, MD, MPH[a],
Rathan M. Subramaniam, MD, PhD, MPH, MBA[b], Lilja B. Solnes, MD, MBA[a],*

KEYWORDS

- [18]F FDG-PET/ CT • Head and neck cancer • Therapy response assessment • Surveillance
- Immunotherapy

KEY POINTS

- Accurate assessment of treatment response and early detection of recurrence in head and neck squamous cell carcinoma (HNSCC) is paramount, allowing for treatment modification and initiation of potentially salvage therapies.
- Radiologists should be aware of the expected posttreatment tissue changes and imaging pitfalls in HNSCC to avoid misinterpretation of studies.
- [18]F FDG-PET/contrast-enhanced CT provides both the metabolic information and high-resolution anatomic detail and is highly sensitive for therapy response assessment in most patients with HNSCC.
- Several ^{18}F FDG-PET-based criteria have been proposed for therapy assessment and surveillance of HNSCC, including the quantitative response criteria (eg, EORTC, PERCIST), and qualitative scoring systems (eg, Hopkins criteria, NI-RADS).

INTRODUCTION

Head and neck cancers are the sixth most common malignancy worldwide with an estimated 450,000 deaths in 2018.[1] Head and neck squamous cell carcinomas (HNSCCs) comprise a diverse group of tumors arising from the oral cavity, oropharynx, hypopharynx, larynx, and nasopharynx.[1] Major risk factors associated with HNSCC are (1) tobacco and alcohol use, which are commonly associated with oral cavity and laryngeal cancers; (2) prior infection with oncogenic strains of human papillomavirus (HPV), mainly associated with oropharyngeal cancers, and (3) Epstein-Barr virus infection in nasopharyngeal cancers.

The incidence of HPV-positive HNSCC has been increasing sharply over the past 2 decades.[2] HPV-positive HNSCCs have distinct clinical presentation, commonly occur in younger age groups, are highly susceptible to chemoradiation therapy, and are associated with longer overall survival.[2]

[a] The Russell H. Morgan Department of Radiology and Radiological Science, Johns Hopkins Medical Institutions, 601 N. Caroline Street, JHOC 3009, Baltimore, MD 21287, USA; [b] Dean's Office, Otago Medical School, University of Otago, 201 Great King Street, Dunedin 9016, New Zealand
* Corresponding author: 601 North Caroline Street, Johns Hopkins Outpatient Center, JHOC # 3009, Baltimore, MD 21287.
E-mail address: lsolnes1@jhmi.edu

PET Clin 17 (2022) 307–317
https://doi.org/10.1016/j.cpet.2021.12.003
1556-8598/22/© 2021 Elsevier Inc. All rights reserved.

Approximately two-thirds of patients with HNSCC present with locally advanced and 10% with metastatic disease.[3] In these patients, multimodality treatments have significantly improved the outcome and quality of life.[4] The principal treatment used for locally advanced HNSCC is surgical resection followed by adjuvant radiotherapy ± platinum-based-chemotherapy, or primary definitive concurrent chemoradiation.[4,5]

Accurate assessment of treatment response and early detection of tumor recurrence before it becomes clinically evident is an essential function of oncologic imaging.[6] Early detection of nonresponders allows modification of the treatment plan, and initiation of potentially salvageable therapeutic strategies. 2-deoxy-2-[^{18}F] fluoro-D-glucose PET/computed tomography (^{18}F FDG-PET/CT) plays a significant role in the staging, therapy assessment, and follow-up of HNSCC.[7] In addition, radiomics signatures and ^{18}F FDG-PET–based imaging biomarkers can provide prognostic information on survival.[8]

This article focuses on the role of ^{18}F-FDG-PET/CT in therapy response assessment of HNSCC; reviews the expected imaging pitfalls after surgery, radiation therapy, and chemotherapy; and discusses common quantitative and qualitative response assessment methods in HNSCC and potential value of imaging surveillance. We also provide an overview of recently approved immune checkpoint inhibitors in HNSCC and common imaging pitfalls in evaluating immunotherapy response.

EXPECTED POSTTREATMENT IMAGING FINDINGS AND INTERPRETIVE PITFALLS

A variety of soft tissue changes can occur following treatment of HNSCC, depending on the type of therapy and site of treatment. Radiologists should be aware of these expected post-therapy tissue changes to avoid misinterpretation of studies as persistent or recurrent disease.[9] Various imaging modalities have been used to assess the posttreatment changes in patients with HNSCC, among which, combined imaging with ^{18}F FDG-PET/CT has been shown to be a highly sensitive modality for evaluation of response, or persistent or recurrent disease in the posttreatment setting, if performed at an appropriate time after therapy.[10]

Expected Tissue Changes After Surgery

Imaging assessment of local recurrence early after surgery can be difficult due to postsurgical anatomic distortion and complexity of the head and neck surgical procedures, reconstruction with pedicle flap, soft tissue flaps, or prosthesis.[9] After major surgery with reconstruction, tumor recurrences usually appear at the edge of the resection or the soft tissue or myocutaneous flaps.[9] Recurrent tumors are more easily identified with ^{18}F FDG-PET/CT than with anatomic imaging alone, due to the increased metabolic activity of recurrent disease. To minimize nontumoral uptake of ^{18}F FDG due to postsurgical inflammation, scarring, and granulation tissue, it is generally recommended that the posttreatment ^{18}F FDG-PET/CT be performed at least 6 weeks after surgery.[11] Occasionally, MR imaging is recommended in patients with sinonasal, nasopharyngeal, and skull base tumors who are at risk for perineural invasion.

Expected Tissue Changes After Radiotherapy

The expected tissue changes after radiotherapy include edema/inflammation in the skin, subcutaneous fat, platysma, and increased enhancement and soft tissue thickening of all the structures in the radiation field, such as pharyngeal walls, laryngeal structures, and major salivary glands.[12] The radiotherapy-induced tissue changes are often symmetric unless the neck is irradiated using asymmetric radiation portals. These changes are most noticeable during the first few months after the completion of radiation therapy, and diminish over time or followed by atrophy of the salivary glands.[9]

False-positive ^{18}F FDG uptake after radiotherapy is commonly caused by radiation-induced mucositis, reactive nodes, soft tissue necrosis, radio-necrosis of bone, and dystrophic calcifications particularly in lymph nodes.[11] To minimize a false-positive result from the postradiation inflammation, it is recommended that posttreatment ^{18}F FDG-PET/CT be performed at least 10 to 12 weeks after completion of radiation therapy.[11]

In addition, post-therapy ^{18}F FDG-PET/CT can improve radiation treatment planning according to the change in tumor volume in response to radiation therapy. In 2016, a multicentric prospective study on 564 patients with HNSCC with advanced nodal disease (stage N2 or N3) who received chemoradiation therapy, showed that ^{18}F FDG-PET/CT-guided surveillance yielded a comparable survival and quality of life relative to planned neck dissection in both HPV-positive and negative patients and is more cost-effective.[13] Absence of FDG uptake at the primary and nodal sites has a high negative predictive value in ruling out residual disease. In patients with HNSCC with residual nodal abnormalities on anatomic imaging after definitive radiation therapy, negative post-therapy ^{18}F FDG-PET/CT can spare neck dissection, particularly in HPV-related oropharyngeal cancer.[14]

Expected Changes After Chemotherapy

In addition to the previously described pitfalls, a number of conditions can occur in patients who received chemotherapy and result in false-positive ^{18}F FDG uptake. Thymic hyperplasia usually occurs in children and young adults at a median of 12 months post chemotherapy and presents with increased ^{18}F FDG uptake in the anterior mediastinum.[11] Intense homogeneous ^{18}F FDG uptake in the bone marrow and spleen can be attributed to granulocyte colony-stimulating factor administration to treat chemotherapy-related neutropenia. Other treatment-related pitfalls/complications include a wide variety of infections due to bone marrow suppression, osteonecrosis, or avascular necrosis.[11]

THERAPY RESPONSE ASSESSMENT: 2-DEOXY-2-[^{18}F] FLUORO-D-GLUCOSE-PET–BASED RESPONSE CRITERIA

A variety of methods have been introduced and standardized to evaluate tumor response to therapy, including the World Health Organization (WHO) in 1981, response evaluation criteria in solid tumors version 1.0 (RECIST) in 2000, and modified RECIST version 1.1 in 2009.[6,12,15] Response evaluation in these anatomic response assessment methods is based on the percentage change in size of target lesions/tumor burden or appearance of new lesions after treatment.[16] The response categorized into 4 groups: complete response; partial response; progressive disease; and stable disease.[12] RECIST 1.1 criteria is the current standard for therapy response assessment in solid tumors in most clinical trials.[16] A detailed review of these anatomic response criteria is beyond the scope of this article.

With increased utilization of ^{18}F FDG-PET/CT in oncology, several ^{18}F FDG-PET-based qualitative and quantitative criteria have been proposed to monitor metabolic changes in response to treatment.[6,12] The first ^{18}F FDG-PET–based criteria attempted to standardize the treatment response was introduced by the European Organization for Research and Treatment of Cancer (EORTC criteria) in 1999.[6] EORTC criteria defined tumor response as a decrease in tumor ^{18}F FDG uptake by 25% or more, and progression as an increase in tumor ^{18}F FDG uptake by more than 25% or the appearance of new lesions.[6] PET Response Criteria in Solid Tumors (PERCIST 1.0) was proposed in 2009, to refine and validate quantitative approaches to assess the metabolic tumor response.[15] Key differences of PERCIST include: (1) the use of standardized uptake values (SUVs)

normalized by lean body mass (SUL) to reduce dependence on patient weight, rather than body surface area in EORTC; (2) use of "SUL peak", measured using a 1-cm^3 fixed-dimension region of interest centered over the area of highest uptake in the tumor instead of mean SUV; (3) Different threshold for tumor response and progression (30% vs 25%), and (4) Different approach to select lesions on the baseline and follow-up scan.[12,15]

Since then, PERCIST has been referenced and incorporated in several clinical trials. PERCIST response categories have been shown to be associated with clinical outcomes after therapy in patients with different types of cancer including HNSCC.[12] A summary of the response categories by EORTC and PERCIST is shown in **Table 1**.

In addition to the quantitative methods, a five-point scale qualitative scoring system, known as the Hopkins criteria, was described in 2014 for therapy response assessment of patients with HNSCC.[17] The Hopkins criteria are qualitative ^{18}F FDG-PET/CT interpretation criteria, scoring the primary tumor and bilateral neck nodal lesions relative to the ^{18}F FDG activity in the internal jugular vein (IJV, reference) and liver as follow; score 1 (Focal uptake less than IJV), score 2 (Focal uptake greater than IJV but less than liver), score 3 (Diffuse uptake greater than IJV or liver), score 4 (Focal uptake greater than liver), score 5 (Focal uptake significantly above liver).[17] Overall scores of 1, 2, and 3 were considered negative for residual disease and scores of 4 and 5 were considered positive for residual disease.[17]

"Hopkins interpretation criteria" has been validated for therapy response assessment of HNSCC in multiple studies including a prospective multi-center study (ECLYPS) on locally advanced patients with HNSCC after concurrent chemoradiotherapy; and a recent phase II randomized trial (NRG HN002) on patients with locally advanced HPV-positive oropharyngeal cancer. Theses studies showed that Hopkins criteria has high negative predictive value (approximately 91.1%-96.5%) for response assessment of primary tumor and nodal disease.[17–19] Hopkins criteria is a reproducible method with moderate to almost perfect inter-reader agreement and can be a predictor of overall survival and progression-free survival in patients with HNSCC and lung cancer.[17–22]

In 2016, the American College of Radiology (ACR) introduced the Neck Imaging Reporting and Data Systems (NI-RADS) as a standardized risk classification system for reporting surveillance imaging of treated patients with HNSCC.[23] NI-RADS was originally designed for surveillance contrast-enhanced CT (CECT) with or without ^{18}F FDG-PET (^{18}F FDG-PET/CECT). In this system,

Table 1
^{18}F FDG-PET–based quantitative and qualitative response criteria for assessment of response to conventional therapies and immunotherapy

Response Assessment Criteria	Complete Metabolic Response (CMR)	Partial Metabolic Response (PMR)	Stable Metabolic Disease (SMD)	Progressive Metabolic Disease (PMD)	Confirmation of Progression
Quantitative Response Assessment					
EORTC (1999)	Tumor no longer identifiable	>25% reduction in SUV after more than one cycle (>15%–25% reduction after 1 cycle of chemotherapy)	Not meeting criteria for CR, PR, PD	≥ 25% increase in SUV; visible increase in extent of uptake or the appearance of new ^{18}F FDG-avid lesions	Not required (unless equivocal)
PERCIST 1.0 (2009)	Complete resolution of uptake of all ^{18}F FDG-avid lesions	≥ 30% reduction in the SULpeak and ≥ 0.8 absolute decrease in SULpeak	Not meeting criteria for CR, PR, PD	≥ 30% increase in SULpeak and an >0.8 absolute increase in SULpeak; new ^{18}F FDG-avid lesions	Not required (unless equivocal)
PERCIMT (2018)	Complete resolution of uptake of all ^{18}F-FDG-avid lesions; no new lesions	Complete resolution of uptake of some ^{18}F-FDG-avid lesions; no new lesions	Not meeting criteria for CR, PR, PD	No clinical benefit Appearance of ≥4 new lesions with functional diameter <1 cm; ≥3 new lesions with functional diameter >1 cm; ≥2 new lesions with functional diameter >1.5 cm	Required (subsequent imaging)
imPERCIST (2019)	Similar to PERCIST 1.0	Similar to PERCIST 1.0	Not meeting criteria for CR, PR, PD	*iUPD:* ≥30% increase in the SULpeak and an >0.8 absolute increase in SULpeak; new ^{18}F FDG-avid lesions *iCPD:* Increase in SULpeak or appearance of new FDG-avid lesions on subsequent examination	Required (subsequent imaging at least 4–8 wk apart)
Qualitative Response Assessment					
Hopkins criteria (2014)	CMR Likely CMR Likely post radiation inflammation Likely residual disease Residual disease	Score 1: Focal FDG uptake less than or equal to IJV Score 2: Focal ^{18}F-FDG uptake greater than IJV but less than liver Score 3: Diffuse ^{18}F-FDG uptake greater than IJV or liver Score 4: Likely residual tumor: Focal ^{18}F-FDG uptake greater than liver Score 5: Focal and intense ^{18}F-FDG uptake greater (2–3 times) than liver			

Abbreviations: IJV, internal jugular vein; SUL, SUVs normalized by lean body mass; SUV, standardized uptake value; PD, progressive disease; PR, partial response; CR, complete response.

the primary tumor, neck lymph nodes, and distant disease (in case of whole-body imaging) are assessed for recurrence and scored based on imaging suspicion (category 0–4) (Figs. 1 and 2). [18]F FDG-PET findings are categorized as no uptake (NI-RADS 1), mild/intermediate uptake (NI-RADS 2) or focal intense uptake (NI-RADS 3). When there is discordance between CT and ^{18}F FDG-PET, the NI-RADS category should be assigned to the lower of the adjacent scores.[23] Table 2 summarizes the NI-RADS category descriptors, imaging findings, and management recommendation.[23]

PROGNOSTIC VALUE OF 2-DEOXY-2-[^{18}F] FLUORO-D-GLUCOSE-PET–BASED METABOLIC PARAMETERS

Visual analysis of ^{18}F FDG-PET/CT is comparable to quantitative assessment and may be adequate for staging and detection of residual disease in HNSCC; however, quantitative evaluation allows a more objective comparison of metabolic activity in the same lesion over time or between patients.[24] Quantitative evaluation is commonly used in the clinical trials as a tool to predict outcome. The commonly studied ^{18}F FDG-PET–based parameters are the standardized uptake value (SUVmax, SUVpeak, SUVmean) and volumetric parameters such as metabolic tumor volume (MTV) and total lesion glycolysis (TLG).[24,25] These functional parameters can be measured on baseline, interim, or post-therapy examinations and have been shown to be independent predictors of early treatment response, progression-free survival, and overall survival in several studies.[24–26] The volumetric parameters are more representative of the heterogeneity of uptake in the tumor and provide higher prognostic value compared with the SUVmax.[24]

A meta-analysis of 26 studies showed that intra-therapy or post-therapy ^{18}F FDG-PET strongly predicts the risk of disease progression and death in patients with HNSCC. A positive ^{18}F FDG-PET result was associated with a more than sixfold increase in the risk of death within 2 years after treatment.[25] [18]F FDG-PET was a better predictor of survival or recurrence when it was performed 12 weeks or more after treatment completion rather than in the interim period.[25]

A recent systematic review on patients with surgically treated HNSCC showed the prognostic effectiveness of preoperative ^{18}F FDG-PET/CT parameters in predicating overall survival, disease-free survival, and distant metastases.[26] The volumetric parameters (MTV and TLG) are particularly useful in identifying patients with a higher risk of postsurgical progression who could receive early

therapeutic intensification to improve their prognosis.[26] The prognostic utility of ^{18}F FDG-PET parameters combined with other predictive biomarkers need to be studied and validated in future studies with larger patient populations.

IMMUNOTHERAPY RESPONSE ASSESSMENT IN HEAD AND NECK CANCER

The introduction of immunotherapy with immune checkpoint inhibitors has changed the landscape of HNSCC therapy, particularly HPV-positive cancers.[5] In 2016, the US Food and Drug Administration approved 2 Programmed death-1 checkpoint inhibitors (anti-PD1), nivolumab and pembrolizumab, for the treatment of recurrent or metastatic HNSCC refractory to platinum-based regimens.[5] In 2019, these agents have been approved for first-line treatment of unresectable or metastatic HNSCC. Pembrolizumab was approved for use in combination with platinum and fluorouracil for all patients and as a single agent for patients whose tumors express PD-L1.[5,27] Immunotherapy has proven to be effective for both HPV-positive and HPV-negative HNSCC.[28] A recent meta-analysis of 1088 patients with HNSCC who received PD-1/L1 inhibitors showed no significant difference on survival or immunotherapy response based on the HPV status.[29]

The pattern of response to immunotherapy is different from cytotoxic chemotherapy, radiotherapy, surgery, and targeted therapies.[12,30] In patients who benefit from immunotherapeutic agents, response seem to be more delayed but durable, due to distinctive biological mechanisms of immune checkpoint inhibitors.[30] In addition, immunotherapy is associated with atypical patterns of response, such as pseudo-progression, dissociative response, prolonged stable disease, and hyper-progression.[31,32] Pseudo-progression is defined as an initial increase in tumor size and/or appearance of new lesions and/or increase in lesion metabolism, followed by subsequent decrease in tumor burden or stabilization of disease.[31] The reported incidence of pseudo-progression is variable in the literature, and can occur in 5% to 15% of metastatic melanoma and approximately 1% of patients with HNSCC.[31,33] Another atypical response pattern is "dissociated response," defined as the coexistence of responding and nonresponding target lesions, and is associated with a better overall survival compared with true progressions.[33] Hyper-progression is defined as a rapid increase in tumor growth kinetics compared with the prior growth rate (at least twofold) and is associated with poor survival outcome.[30]

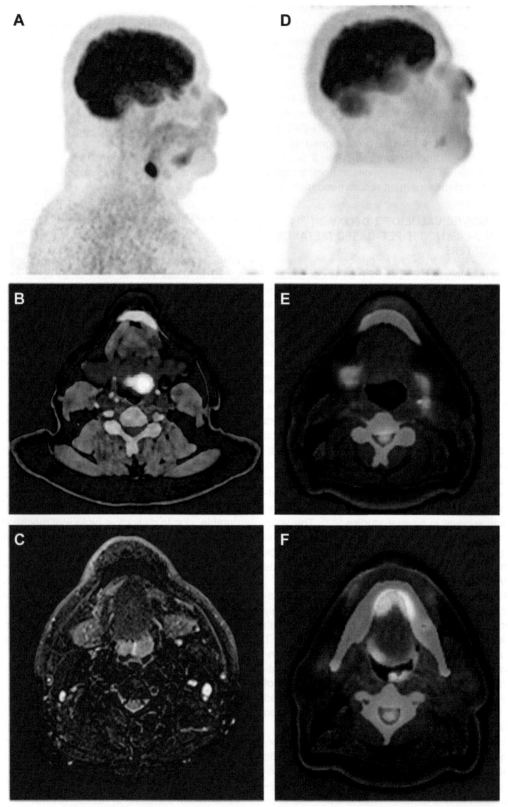

Fig. 1. A 58-year-old man with HPV 16-positive squamous cell carcinoma of the left lingual tonsil. Staging ^{18}F FDG-PET/CT (*A*, *B*) and neck MR imaging (axial short tau inversion recovery; *C*) showed intensely hypermetabolic mass at base of the tongue/left lingual tonsil with no evidence of adenopathy or distant metastases. Follow-up ^{18}F FDG-PET/CT after neoadjuvant immunotherapy and surgical resection (*D–F*), showed mild inflammatory up-take in the posterior oropharynx (*F*), and complete metabolic resolution of primary tumor with no evidence of recurrent disease (Hopkins criteria-score 1; NI-RADS category 1).

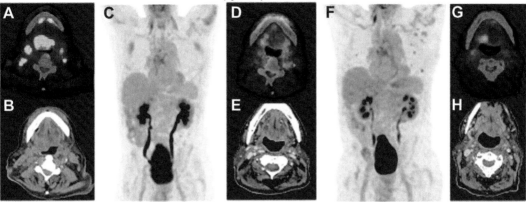

Fig. 2. A 78-year-old man with HPV-positive squamous cell carcinoma of the right base of the tongue with bilateral cervical adenopathy (T3N2bM0) on staging ^{18}F FDG-PET/CT (*A, B*). ^{18}F FDG-PET/CT after completion of chemoradiation therapy (*C–E*) showed complete metabolic resolution of primary tumor and cervical adenopathy without evidence of metastases (NI-RADS category 1). Follow-up ^{18}F FDG-PET/CT, 8 months posttreatment, showed new non–mass-like soft tissue thickening at the right base of the tongue with mild differential enhancement and mild ^{18}F FDG uptake (NI-RADS score 2b), and multiple new ^{18}F FDG-avid pulmonary nodules (NI-RADS score 4). Findings are consistent with progression to metastatic disease.

Table 2
ACR NI-RADS categories and management recommendations for surveillance of head and neck squamous cell carcinomas

		Imaging Findings		
	Category	Contrast-Enhanced Computed Tomography	^{18}F FDG-PET	Management Recommendation
0	Incomplete Assessment	New Baseline Study with No Prior Imaging Available		Obtain Prior Imaging Examinations
1	No evidence of recurrence	Non–mass-like distortion of soft tissues Mild mucoid" mucosal edema or diffuse linear mucosal enhancement post radiation	No abnormal FDG uptake	Routine surveillance
2a	Low suspicion	Non–mass-like, focal, mucosal enhancement	Focal mild to moderate FDG uptake	Direct visual inspection
2b		Non–mass-like, ill-defined, deep soft tissue with only minimal differential enhancement Residual abnormal node(s), without new suspicious morphology		Short-interval follow-up (3 mo), repeat PET
3	High suspicion	New or enlarging primary mass or lymph node Discrete nodule/mass with differential enhancement Enlarging node(s), with new necrosis or gross extranodal extension	Intense focal FDG uptake	Image guided or clinical biopsy
4	Definite recurrence	Pathologically proven or definite radiologic and clinical progression		Clinical management

The main difference in evaluation of response to immunotherapy compared with other treatments is in the classification of progressive disease. Progressive disease requires confirmation on 2 consecutive imaging assessments at least 4 weeks apart to exclude pseudo-progression.[30] The inaccurate interpretation of immunotherapy response can result in premature termination of potentially beneficial therapy. Thus, the clinical status and stability should be considered to guide therapeutic decisions in patients with unconfirmed progressive disease.[30]

A series of modified immune-related criteria have been proposed for immunotherapy response assessment, including the immune-related response criteria (irRC, 2009, adapted from the WHO criteria); immune-related RECIST (irRECIST, introduced in 2014); immune-modified RECIST (imRECIST, 2018), and the immune RECIST (iRECIST, 2017).[30] The proposed ^{18}F FDG-PET–based response assessment criteria include PET response evaluation criteria for immunotherapy (PERCIMT, 2018), and immunotherapy-modified PERCIST (imPERCIST, 2019), summarized in **Table 1**.[14,34,35]

The Society for Immunotherapy of Cancer Head and Neck Cancer subcommittee, established an evidence-based consensus guideline on emerging application of immunotherapies for treatment of patients with HNSCC.[5] Key recommendations were focused on appropriate patient selection, response monitoring, adverse event management, and biomarker testing.[5] Herein, we briefly discuss the recommended guideline on immunotherapy response monitoring.[5]

Initial assessment: The subcommittee recommends using either a CT (53%) or ^{18}F FDG-PET/CT (41%) following a baseline clinical examination.

Response assessment method: Most immunotherapy clinical trials used RECIST v1.1 to assess the efficacy of anti-PD1 therapy. Thus, the subcommittee was split in their recommendation of RECIST v1.1 (56%) versus irRECIST (44%) to assess the immunotherapy response in patients with HNSCC. There is still no consensus on the optimal timeframe and interval for immunotherapy response assessment. However, most of the subcommittee (65%) recommends standard of care imaging evaluation every 3 months after initial follow-up to monitor signs of response.

Determining duration of treatment: In patients with complete or near-complete immunotherapy response, the current consensus is to continue treatment for at least 1 or 2 years or until disease progression or toxicity. In patients with early radiographic progression who are clinically stable, the consensus is to continue treatment until progression is confirmed on a second scan. If a patient has symptomatic progression/clinical deterioration, the treatment should stop.

Identification of immune-related symptoms and adverse events: Patients need to be evaluated at least monthly, and sometimes more frequently in the setting of active adverse events.

SURVEILLANCE STRATEGIES IN HEAD AND NECK CANCER

Posttreatment surveillance is an important component of HNSCC management. Locoregional recurrence may be seen in up to 48% of patients with HNSCC, depending on the primary site, initial staging, and treatment modality. Most recurrences tend to occur within the first 2 years after treatment. Recent studies highlighted the different pattern of disease progression in HNSCC based on HPV status. In HPV-positive patients, distant metastases may occur later and in unexpected sites.[36]

Effective surveillance allows early detection of tumor recurrence, or second primary malignancy (eg, lung cancer) and will increase success and minimize the toxicity of salvage treatment. Traditionally, surveillance in HNSCC includes clinical examination, performed every 3 to 4 months in the first 2 years, every 4 to 6 months in years 2 to 5, and then annually. Surveillance imaging has been increasingly performed for the detection of tumor recurrence in patients with HNSCC, using various modalities, including CT, ^{18}F FDG-PET, and MR imaging. [18]F FDG-PET/contrast-enhanced CT has been adopted as the imaging of choice for therapy response assessment in most patients with HNSCC, as it can provide both the metabolic information and high-resolution anatomic detail.[23] Follow-up ^{18}F FDG-PET/CT, performed 4 months or later after completion of treatment, has been shown to have superior performance for recurrence detection compared with anatomic imaging, including CT or MRI alone.[37] A meta-analysis of 23 studies, including 2247 examinations showed a pooled sensitivity and specificity of 92% and 87% for follow-up ^{18}F FDG-PET/CT in curatively treated patients with HNSCC.[38] Subgroup analysis based on the time of follow-up examination showed higher specificity (91% vs 78%) and comparable sensitivity for ^{18}F FDG-PET/CT, when performed ≥12 months compared with 4 to 12 months after completion of treatment.[38] Despite this promising result, the routine use of ^{18}F FDG-PET/CT is not recommended in long-term surveillance of HNSCC, unless there is clinical suspicion of recurrence or prior equivocal imaging finding.

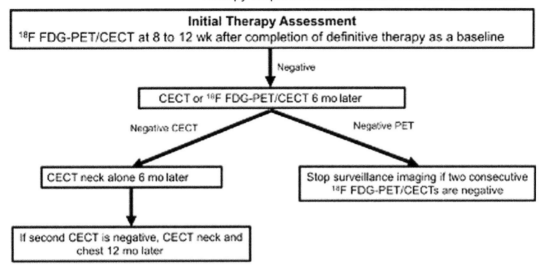

Fig. 3. ACR NI-RADS proposed surveillance imaging algorithm for posttreatment assessment of head and neck cancers.

There is variability in the HNSCC surveillance strategies in different institutions. The National Comprehensive Cancer Network guidelines in head and neck cancer recommend imaging within the first 6 months following treatment completion. No official recommendation for surveillance imaging beyond 6 months in asymptomatic patients with HNSCC exists. To address this shortcoming, ACR NI-RADS proposed a standard posttreatment surveillance imaging algorithm for HNSCC, which is depicted in **Fig. 3**.[23]

Given the scarcity of evidence supporting the proposed surveillance or imaging strategies, surveillance methods should be tailored at each institution and clinical judgment should be used to decide on the optimal surveillance plan for each individual patient.[37] Future studies are needed to compare the performance, cost-effectiveness, and prognostic value of different surveillance strategies to determine the frequency and optimal modality for long-term surveillance of HNSCC.

SUMMARY

18F FDG-PET/CT has been shown to be a highly sensitive modality for evaluation of treatment response, early detection of persistent or recurrent disease, or second primary tumors in the post-treatment setting, if performed at the appropriate time after therapy. Several 18F FDG-PET–based quantitative and qualitative methods have been shown to be effective for therapy response assessment and surveillance of HNSCC. There is variability in the HNSCC surveillance strategies in different institutions and no consensus recommendation on the effectiveness and survival benefit of surveillance imaging beyond 6 months in asymptomatic patients with HNSCC exists.

CLINICS CARE POINTS

- To be able differentiate residual tumor from findings related to postsurgical/post-radiation inflammation and scaring, it is generally recommended that the post-treatment 18F FDG-PET/CT be performed at least 6 weeks after surgery and 10 to 12 weeks after completion of radiation therapy.

- The "Hopkins criteria", is a qualitative interpretation system, scoring the primary tumor and bilateral neck nodal lesions relative to the 18F FDG activity in the internal jugular vein (IJV, reference) and liver; and has been validated for HNSCC therapy response assessment in multiple studies.

- The Neck Imaging Reporting and Data Systems (NI-RADS) is a standardized risk classification method for reporting surveillance CECT and/or PET/CECT imaging in HNSCC. In this system, the primary tumor, neck lymph nodes, and distant disease are scored based on imaging suspicion for recurrence (category 0–4).

- Immunotherapy has proven to be effective for both HPV-positive and HPV-negative HNSCC. In patients with complete or near-complete response, treatment can be continued for at least 1 or 2 years or until disease progression or toxicity. In patients with early radiographic progression who are clinically stable, the consensus is to continue immunotherapy treatment until progression is confirmed on a second scan.

DISCLOSURE

None.

REFERENCES

1. Johnson DE, Burtness B, Leemans CR, et al. Head and neck squamous cell carcinoma. Nat Rev Dis Primers 2020;6:92.
2. Pan C, Issaeva N, Yarbrough WG. HPV-driven oropharyngeal cancer: current knowledge of molecular biology and mechanisms of carcinogenesis. Cancers Head Neck 2018;3:12.
3. Denaro N, Merlano MC, Russi EG. Follow-up in head and neck cancer: do more does it mean do better? A systematic review and our proposal based on our experience. Clin Exp Otorhinolaryngol 2016;9:287–97.
4. Cognetti DM, Weber RS, Lai SY. Head and neck cancer: an evolving treatment paradigm. Cancer 2008;113:1911–32.
5. Cohen EEW, Bell RB, Bifulco CB, et al. The Society for Immunotherapy of Cancer consensus statement on immunotherapy for the treatment of squamous cell carcinoma of the head and neck (HNSCC). J Immunother Cancer 2019;7:184.
6. Sheikhbahaei S, Mena E, Pattanayak P, et al. Molecular imaging and precision medicine: PET/computed tomography and therapy response assessment in oncology. PET Clin 2017;12:105–18.
7. Pfister DG, Spencer S, Adelstein D, et al. Head and neck cancers, version 2.2020, NCCN clinical practice guidelines in oncology. J Natl Compr Canc Netw 2020;18:873–98.
8. Martens RM, Koopman T, Noij DP, et al. Predictive value of quantitative (18)F-FDG-PET radiomics analysis in patients with head and neck squamous cell carcinoma. EJNMMI Res 2020;10:102.
9. Saito N, Nadgir RN, Nakahira M, et al. Posttreatment CT and MR imaging in head and neck cancer: what the radiologist needs to know. Radiographics 2012;32:1261–82.
10. Kostakoglu L, Goldsmith SJ. PET in the assessment of therapy response in patients with carcinoma of the head and neck and of the esophagus. J Nucl Med 2004;45:56–68.
11. Long NM, Smith CS. Causes and imaging features of false positives and false negatives on F-PET/CT in oncologic imaging. Insights Imaging 2011;2:679–98.
12. Tirkes T, Hollar MA, Tann M, et al. Response criteria in oncologic imaging: review of traditional and new criteria. Radiographics 2013;33:1323–41.
13. Mehanna H, Wong WL, McConkey CC, et al. PET-CT surveillance versus neck dissection in advanced head and neck cancer. N Engl J Med 2016;374:1444–54.
14. Kishikawa T, Suzuki M, Takemoto N, et al. Response Evaluation Criteria in Solid Tumors (RECIST) and PET Response Criteria in Solid Tumors (PERCIST) for response evaluation of the neck after chemoradiotherapy in head and neck squamous cell carcinoma. Head Neck 2021;43:1184–93.
15. Wahl RL, Jacene H, Kasamon Y, et al. From RECIST to PERCIST: evolving considerations for PET response criteria in solid tumors. J Nucl Med 2009;50(Suppl 1):122S–50S.
16. Yaghmai V, Miller FH, Rezai P, et al. Response to treatment series: part 2, tumor response assessment–using new and conventional criteria. AJR Am J Roentgenol 2011;197:18–27.
17. Marcus C, Ciarallo A, Tahari AK, et al. Head and neck PET/CT: therapy response interpretation criteria (Hopkins Criteria)-interreader reliability, accuracy, and survival outcomes. J Nucl Med 2014;55:1411–6.
18. Kendi AT, Brandon D, Switchenko J, et al. Head and neck PET/CT therapy response interpretation criteria (Hopkins criteria) - external validation study. Am J Nucl Med Mol Imaging 2017;7:174–80.
19. Van den Wyngaert T, Helsen N, Carp L, et al. Fluorodeoxyglucose-positron emission tomography/computed tomography after concurrent chemoradiotherapy in locally advanced head-and-neck squamous cell cancer: the ECLYPS study. J Clin Oncol 2017;35:3458–64.
20. Sheikhbahaei S, Mena E, Marcus C, et al. 18F-FDG PET/CT: therapy response assessment interpretation (Hopkins criteria) and survival outcomes in lung cancer patients. J Nucl Med 2016;57:855–60.
21. Helsen N, Van den Wyngaert T, Carp L, et al. Quantification of 18F-fluorodeoxyglucose uptake to detect residual nodal disease in locally advanced head and neck squamous cell carcinoma after chemoradiotherapy: results from the ECLYPS study. Eur J Nucl Med Mol Imaging 2020;47:1075–82.
22. Zhong J, Sundersingh M, Dyker K, et al. Post-treatment FDG PET-CT in head and neck carcinoma: comparative analysis of 4 qualitative interpretative criteria in a large patient cohort. Sci Rep 2020;10:4086.
23. Aiken AH, Rath TJ, Anzai Y, et al. ACR neck imaging reporting and data systems (NI-RADS): a white paper of the ACR NI-RADS Committee. J Am Coll Radiol 2018;15:1097–108.
24. Paterson C, Hargreaves S, Rumley CN. Functional imaging to predict treatment response in head and neck cancer: how close are we to biologically adaptive radiotherapy? Clin Oncol (R Coll Radiol 2020;32:861–73.
25. Sheikhbahaei S, Ahn SJ, Moriarty E, et al. Intratherapy or posttherapy FDG PET or FDG PET/CT for patients with head and neck cancer: a systematic review and meta-analysis of prognostic studies. AJR Am J Roentgenol 2015;205:1102–13.
26. Creff G, Devillers A, Depeursinge A, et al. Evaluation of the prognostic value of FDG PET/CT parameters

for patients with surgically treated head and neck cancer: a systematic review. JAMA Otolaryngol Head Neck Surg 2020;146:471–9.

27. FDA approves pembrolizumab for first-line treatment of head and neck squamous cell carcinoma. Available at: https://www.fda.gov/drugs/resources-infor mation-approved-drugs/fda-approves-pembrolizu mab-first-line-treatment-head-and-neck-squamous-cell-carcinoma. Accessed July 15th, 2021.

28. Carlisle JW, Steuer CE, Owonikoko TK, et al. An update on the immune landscape in lung and head and neck cancers. CA Cancer J Clin 2020;70:505–17.

29. Patel JJ, Levy DA, Nguyen SA, et al. Impact of PD-L1 expression and human papillomavirus status in anti-PD1/PDL1 immunotherapy for head and neck squamous cell carcinoma-systematic review and meta-analysis. Head Neck 2020;42:774–86.

30. Nishino M, Hatabu H, Hodi FS. Imaging of cancer immunotherapy: current approaches and future directions. Radiology 2019;290:9–22.

31. Borcoman E, Kanjanapan Y, Champiat S, et al. Novel patterns of response under immunotherapy. Ann Oncol 2019;30:385–96.

32. Lauber K, Dunn L. Immunotherapy mythbusters in head and neck cancer: the abscopal effect and pseudoprogression. Am Soc Clin Oncol Educ Book 2019;39:352–63.

33. Sheikhbahaei S, Verde F, Hales RK, et al. Imaging in therapy response assessment and surveillance of lung cancer: evidenced-based review with focus on the utility of (18)F-FDG PET/CT. Clin Lung Cancer 2020;21:485–97.

34. Anwar H, Sachpekidis C, Winkler J, et al. Absolute number of new lesions on (18)F-FDG PET/CT is more predictive of clinical response than SUV changes in metastatic melanoma patients receiving ipilimumab. Eur J Nucl Med Mol Imaging 2018;45:376–83.

35. Goldfarb L, Duchemann B, Chouahnia K, et al. Monitoring anti-PD-1-based immunotherapy in non-small cell lung cancer with FDG PET: introduction of iPER-CIST. EJNMMI Res 2019;9:8.

36. Benjamin J, Hephzibah J, Shanthly N, et al. F-18 FDG PET-CT for response evaluation in head and neck malignancy: experience from a tertiary level hospital in south India. Cancer Rep (Hoboken) 2021;4:e1333.

37. Zhao X, Rao S. Surveillance imaging following treatment of head and neck cancer. Semin Oncol 2017;44:323–9.

38. Sheikhbahaei S, Taghipour M, Ahmad R, et al. Diagnostic accuracy of follow-up FDG PET or PET/CT in patients with head and neck cancer after definitive treatment: a systematic review and meta-analysis. AJR Am J Roentgenol 2015;205:629–39.

PET/Computed Tomography

Post-therapy Follow-up in Head and Neck Cancer

Helena You, MD[a],*, Rathan M. Subramaniam, MD, PhD, MPH, MBA[b,c]

KEYWORDS

- ^{18}F-FDG • PET/CT • Head and neck cancer • Follow-up • Surveillance

KEY POINTS

- PET/computed tomography (CT) plays an important role in post-therapy follow-up of head and neck cancer patients and is sensitive in detecting recurrence and metastasis.
- Baseline post-therapy PET/CT should be performed within 3 months to 6 months after completion of definitive treatment and no earlier than 12 weeks to reduce false-positive results.
- There is limited benefit of routine follow-up PET/CT in asymptomatic patients with a negative baseline PET/CT at 3 months post-therapy. If follow-up PET/CT is performed, yield may be higher earlier in the post-therapy period, although in the subgroup of human papillomavirus (HPV)-related tumors, recurrences tend to occur later in the disease course.
- Additional post-therapy PET/CT imaging should be individualized to patients based on considerations such as tumor type, stage, prognostic factors, symptoms, and clinical assessment.
- Liquid biopsy with biomarkers, such as circulating or salivary HPV DNA, shows potential for complementing PET/CT in detecting recurrence of HPV-related tumors.

INTRODUCTION

Head and neck cancers represent approximately 4% of all cancers in the United States and the sixth most common cancer worldwide.[1,2] In 2020, there were more than 53,000 estimated new cases of oropharyngeal cancers and more than 10,000 estimated deaths due to oropharyngeal cancers in the United States.[1] These cancers typically arise from squamous epithelium of the oral cavity, pharynx, or larynx. Incidence and mortality rates of head and neck cancers, in particular, oropharyngeal squamous cell carcinomas (OPSCCs), have been on the rise owing to increasing human papillomavirus (HPV)-related cancers.[3] Treatment of head and neck cancers frequently is multimodal and includes surgery, chemotherapy, and radiation therapy as well as targeted therapies and immune checkpoint inhibitors, pembrolizumab and nivolumab.[4,5]

[18]F-fluorodeoxyglucose (FDG) PET/computed tomography (CT) can be utilized in initial staging of head and neck cancers, assessing treatment response, and detecting recurrence and metastases.[6,7] Increasingly, PET/CT has been utilized in addition to anatomic imaging with CT and MR imaging for initial staging and as a replacement for CT and MR imaging in post-therapy follow-up of head and neck cancers.[8] Studies have demonstrated the utility of PET/CT for detecting recurrence of head and neck cancers and predicting survival outcomes.[9,10] Post-treatment PET/CT has been shown to have an impact on patient management as well.[11,12] In patients with

[a] Department of Radiology, Stanford University School of Medicine, 300 Pasteur Drive, Suite H1330, Stanford, CA 94305, USA; [b] Dean's Office, Otago Medical School, University of Otago, Dunedin 9016, New Zealand; [c] Department of Radiology, Duke University, Durham, NC 27705, USA
* Corresponding author.
E-mail address: helena.you@stanford.edu

PET Clin 17 (2022) 319–326
https://doi.org/10.1016/j.cpet.2021.12.001

advanced nodal disease who have negative post-therapy PET/CT, planned neck dissection can be avoided because PET/CT surveillance has comparable survival and quality of life to neck dissection while being more cost-effective.[13]

National Comprehensive Cancer Network (NCCN) guidelines for head and neck cancer provide recommendations for post-therapy imaging follow-up in addition to routine clinical assessment. Follow-up PET/CT is recommended between 3 months and 6 months after completion of definitive therapy and no sooner than 12 weeks post-therapy in order to reduce false-positive results.[14] After this initial post-therapy PET/CT imaging, there is an unclear role for further routine imaging surveillance of asymptomatic patients. This article aims to provide an overview of post-therapy follow-up of head and neck cancers with a focus on the role of PET/CT imaging. In this discussion, post-therapy follow-up PET/CT is defined as PET/CT performed after 6 months of therapy completion, because NCCN guidelines recommend a therapy assessment scan (referred to as baseline post-therapy PET/CT in this discussion) between 3 months and 6 months after therapy completion.

OVERVIEW OF POST-THERAPY FOLLOW-UP

Following definitive treatment of head and neck cancers, follow-up is an essential part of continued patient care. Post-therapy follow-up serves multiple purposes, including evaluation of response to therapy, detection of recurrent or metastatic disease, and assessment for therapy-related complications. Clinical assessment and imaging are used in conjunction, and both are important components of post-therapy follow-up.

Clinical Assessment

Head and neck cancer patients typically are followed for at least several years following completion of definitive therapy. At follow-up visits, patients are assessed clinically with a history and physical examination, including a complete head and neck examination as well as mirror and fiberoptic examinations. History is elicited from the patient to determine the presence of any signs or symptoms concerning for disease recurrence. A comprehensive head and neck examination also is performed, which includes indirect mirror examination and fiberoptic nasopharyngolaryngoscopy for most patients in order to fully evaluate the site of the tumor.[15]

The frequency of routine follow-up visits typically is highest early in the post-therapy period and gradually tapers with time from treatment. NCCN guidelines suggest clinical follow-up every 1 month to 3 months in the first post-therapy year, every 2 months to 6 months in the second year, every 4 months to 8 months in years 3 to 5, and then spaced out to yearly after 5 years.[14] Clinical follow-up involves a multidisciplinary approach, frequently involving the input of ear, nose, and throat physicians; medical and radiation oncologists; dentists; dietitians; speech therapists; and radiologists.[15]

Imaging and Role of PET/Computed Tomography

Imaging plays an essential role in post-therapy follow-up of head and neck cancers. Multiple imaging modalities, including CT, MR imaging, PET/CT, and ultrasound, can be used in post-therapy imaging follow-up, each with its own benefits and limitations.

Increasingly, PET/CT has become a preferred modality for post-therapy follow-up imaging given its utility in detecting local, regional, and distant disease. A recent meta-analysis of 26 studies by Sheikhbahaei and colleagues[16] reported high diagnostic performance of PET/CT in detecting recurrent disease, with a pooled sensitivity of 92% and specificity of 87%. Previous meta-analyses reported similar estimates of sensitivity and specificity. For example, an earlier meta-analysis by Gupta and colleagues[10] reported a pooled sensitivity of 91.9% and specificity of 86.9% for the primary site and a pooled sensitivity of 90.4% and specificity of 94.3% for neck nodes when PET/CT was performed more than 12 weeks post-therapy. A meta-analysis by Gao and colleagues[17] similarly reported a sensitivity of 92% and specificity of 95% for detecting distant metastatic disease before salvage treatment in patients with suspected recurrent head and neck cancer.

Post-therapy PET/CT is useful in detecting recurrence that otherwise may be missed on routine clinical examination or conventional imaging. A prospective study by Kim and colleagues[9] found that PET/CT was more sensitive than conventional imaging with CT or MR imaging and also detected 65 of 66 (98.5%) recurrences that were not suggested by physical examination and endoscopy during regular clinical follow-up. Furthermore, PET/CT can have an impact on patient management and predict survival. A prospective study by Krabbe and colleagues[18] found post-therapy PET/CT for oral cavity and oropharyngeal cancer was more sensitive for recurrence than regular clinical follow-up and also led to more changes in diagnostic procedures or treatment. Similarly, Kostakoglu and colleagues[12] found

PET/CT to detect more recurrences than CT or clinical assessment with physical examination and endoscopy and also led to significant change in management.

NATIONAL COMPREHENSIVE CANCER NETWORK GUIDELINES FOR POST-THERAPY IMAGING

The NCCN provides guidelines for follow-up imaging of head and neck cancers in the short term (less than 6 months post-therapy) and long term (6 months to 5 years post-therapy). After definitive treatment of head and neck cancer, anatomic imaging with CT or MR imaging typically is performed within 3 months to 4 months after therapy to establish a new baseline for future follow-up imaging. If there is concern for incomplete therapy response, CT or MR imaging may be performed even earlier. Ultrasound also may be utilized, particularly for evaluation of the neck and for sampling of suspected nodal disease.[14]

For PET/CT, however, NCCN guidelines recommend imaging no earlier than 12 weeks after completion of definitive therapy in order to reduce false-positive results related to inflammatory changes or slow responding tumors that have may positive FDG uptake but negative results at biopsy.[14,16,19,20] Thus, follow-up PET/CT imaging is recommended within 3 months to 6 months after definitive therapy to assess response as well as to identify residual disease.[14,18,21] The ECLYPS study, a prospective multicenter study on follow-up PET/CT after chemoradiation therapy for locally advanced head and neck squamous cell cancer (HNSCC), found PET/CT identified recurrent disease with gradually decreasing sensitivity with increasing time after initial post-therapy imaging at 12 weeks. In this study, PET/CT had high sensitivity up to 9 months after initial post-therapy imaging.[22] A negative post-therapy PET/CT within 6 months after treatment has significant prognostic value. Kao and colleagues[23] found that 2-year progression-free survival and overall survival rates were significantly higher in patients with a negative PET/CT within 6 months after completion of radiation therapy.

ROUTINE POST-THERAPY PET/COMPUTED TOMOGRAPHY AND TIMING IN ASYMPTOMATIC PATIENTS

Most recurrences of head and neck cancer occur within the first 2 years after treatment.[24,25] Beswick and colleagues[24] found that 45% of asymptomatic recurrences of HNSCC were detected within the first 6 months after treatment, 79%

within the first 12 months, 95% within the first 24 months, and 100% within 48 months. Thus, it can be reasoned that the yield of additional imaging is higher when performed earlier in the post-therapy time period. McDermott and colleagues[26] found that 2 consecutive negative PET/CTs within 6 months post-therapy had 98% negative predictive value (NPV) and could obviate further routine follow-up imaging in asymptomatic patients.

After the initial baseline PET/CT at 3 months to 6 months post-therapy, however, further routine imaging is of unclear benefit in an asymptomatic patient with a negative scan. Ho and colleagues[27] evaluated the impact of routine PET/CT imaging at 12 months and 24 months post-therapy in patients with an initial negative scan at 3 months. Detection rates for locoregional recurrence were low at 2% and 0% at 12 months and 24 months, respectively. For distant metastasis, detection rates were slightly higher, at 6% and 4%, at 12 and 24 months, respectively. There was no significant difference, however, in disease-free survival or overall survival rates at 3 years in patients with PET/CT-detected versus clinically detected recurrence.[27] Thus, even if routine surveillance PET/CT detects asymptomatic recurrence, there is unclear impact on survival.

In concordance with these findings, NCCN guidelines recommend against routine imaging in patients with a negative PET/CT at 3 months post-therapy and negative clinical examination, with additional imaging indicated for those with worrisome or equivocal signs and symptoms. NCCN guidelines also state that routine surveillance imaging can be considered to visualize areas that are inaccessible on clinical examination, such as anatomic locations that are deep-seated or obscured by treatment-related changes. Overall, the approach to routine post-therapy surveillance imaging should be individualized to patients based on considerations, such as tumor type, stage, prognostic factors, symptoms, and clinical assessment.[14]

POST-THERAPY FOLLOW-UP IN HUMAN PAPILLOMAVIRUS–RELATED CANCERS

Although head and neck cancers traditionally are associated with the risk factors of tobacco and alcohol use, increasing infections with high-risk HPV strains have led to a rise in HPV-related head and neck cancers.[28] HPV-positive cancers are clinically distinct from HPV-negative cancers and tend to have more favorable therapy response and survival outcomes.[29–31] Additionally, HPV-positive cancers tend to have longer time to recurrence and metastasize to unusual distant sites, such as liver, bone, and brain.[31–34]

NCCN guidelines for post-therapy imaging of head and neck cancers do not distinguish between HPV-positive and HPV-negative disease. In both HPV-positive and HPV-negative advanced HNSCC, Mehanna and colleagues[13] found PET/CT surveillance at 12 weeks post-therapy to be noninferior to planned neck dissection. PET/CT has been reported, however, to have lower diagnostic performance in HPV-positive compared with HPV-negative disease and often may have equivocal findings, with several studies having reported low positive predictive values (PPVs) for the baseline post-therapy PET/CT in HPV-positive patients.[35–39] Liu and colleagues[40] evaluated the utility of a repeat PET/CT at 16 weeks post-therapy after an initial baseline post-therapy PET/CT at 12 weeks, instead of neck dissection, in patients with HPV-positive OPSCC who had incomplete nodal response after therapy. Approximately 71% of patients with incomplete response at 12 weeks converted to complete response at 16 weeks and avoided neck dissection. PPV of the 16-week PET/CT, however, still was low, at 33%, although higher than the 12-week PET/CT PPV of 12%.[40]

The value of additional post-therapy PET/CT follow-up of HPV-related cancers in the longer term is unclear. Given the more favorable prognosis of HPV-related disease, there may be even more limited benefit in follow-up imaging of asymptomatic HPV-positive patients. For example, Corpman and colleagues[36] evaluated follow-up surveillance PET/CT performed beyond 26 weeks post-therapy in HPV-positive OPSCCs. These follow-up PET/CT scans were found to have 100% sensitivity and NPV but lower specificity of 72.4% and PPV of only 8.1%. Although the follow-up PET/CTs led to 22 additional imaging studies and 8 biopsies, none of the 126 follow-up PET/CTs led to meaningful salvage therapy. The investigators also found no survival difference between clinically detected and PET/CT-detected recurrence.[36] On the other hand, HPV-positive cancers tend to take a longer period to recur and may present with distant metastases that would be difficult to appreciate on clinical examination. These characteristics could suggest a longer time period of post-therapy follow-up at perhaps a decreased intensity. A small study by Su and colleagues[41] found HPV-related OPSCC to recur at a median 19.7 months from treatment completion, compared with 11.5 months for the HPV-negative group, with 12 of 16 asymptomatic recurrences detected by PET/CT alone, supporting a potential role for continued imaging surveillance for this patient population.

LIQUID BIOPSY IN POST-THERAPY FOLLOW-UP

Liquid biopsy, which broadly refers to the detection of biomarkers in body fluid specimens to detect, characterize, and monitor tumor burden, offers a rapid, noninvasive method of identifying tumor recurrence or metastasis.[42,43] In head and neck cancers, liquid biopsy can be performed with either blood or salivary specimens. Circulating cell-free HPV DNA is one such biomarker that is found in patients with HPV-related head and neck cancers.[44] A recent meta-analysis by Wuerdemann and colleagues[45] reported a pooled sensitivity of 73% and specificity of 100% of circulating HPV DNA for follow-up of HPV-positive HNSCC, similar to a prior meta-analysis by Jensen and colleagues[45,46] that also reported high specificity but moderate sensitivity.[46] Ahn and colleagues[47] found HPV DNA detection to be more sensitive in plasma (55.1%) compared with saliva (18.8%), whereas the combination of plasma and saliva HPV DNA was even more sensitive, at 69.5%. Specificity remained high (over 90%) with each method.[47]

Other strategies for liquid biopsy in post-therapy follow-up that have been suggested in studies include the use of consecutive HPV DNA testing as well as HPV DNA as a complement to PET/CT. Chera and colleagues[48] found detection of circulating HPV DNA in 2 consecutive plasma samples, 6 months to 9 months apart, to have high PPV (94%) and NPV (100%) for identifying recurrent disease in HPV-positive OPSCC. The investigators suggested that performing PET/CT in patients who have 2 consecutive positive HPV DNA tests may be a potentially cost-effective strategy for identifying recurrence.[48]

In comparing liquid biopsy to imaging follow-up, Tanaka and colleagues[49] found circulating HPV DNA and PET/CT to have similar NPV (89.7% compared with 84.0%, respectively), whereas PPV was much higher with HPV DNA (100% compared with 50%, respectively). Lee and colleagues[50] found circulating HPV DNA levels to correlate well with clinical response. The investigators noted that of 3 patients with increased FDG uptake at the primary site on baseline post-therapy PET/CT but negative HPV DNA levels, none had positive biopsy findings and all had complete resolution of disease on subsequent PET/CT.[50] Similarly, Rutkowski and colleagues[51] found that in 23 patients with incomplete radiologic response on baseline post-therapy PET/CT or MR imaging, only those with residual circulating HPV DNA levels had treatment failure, whereas those with negative HPV DNA levels had complete resolution of disease on subsequent examination.[51] These studies suggest a complementary role of liquid biopsy with HPV DNA and PET/CT in follow-up of HPV-positive head and neck cancers.

IMMUNOTHERAPY FOR HEAD AND NECK CANCERS

Recently, immunotherapy has emerged as an important development in the management of head and neck cancers. Immune checkpoint inhibitors, such as programmed cell death protein 1 (PD-1) inhibitors, target T-cell activation pathways in order to mount an antitumor immune response.[52] PD-1 inhibitors pembrolizumab and nivolumab were first approved by the US Food and Drug Administration (FDA) for recurrent or metastatic HNSCC in patients with disease progression despite standard-of-care treatment with chemotherapy. In 2019, pembrolizumab also was approved by the FDA as first-line treatment of patients with metastatic or unresectable recurrent HNSCC based on the KEYNOTE-048 study, which established the efficacy of pembrolizumab, with or without chemotherapy, for this patient population.[5]

Patterns of therapy response to immunotherapy can differ from those to chemoradiation. For example, pseudoprogression refers to initial signs of progression followed by response, which may be due to immune cell infiltration of the tumor or delayed response. Hyperprogression is another phenomenon, in which there is acceleration of tumor growth after receiving immunotherapy.[53,54] Subsequently, response metrics specific to immunotherapy have been developed, such as immune-related Response Evaluation Criteria in Solid Tumors and PET/CT Criteria for Early Prediction of Response to Immune Checkpoint Inhibitor Therapy.[54,55] Currently, there is a lack of data on post-therapy follow-up PET/CT in HNSCC patients treated with immunotherapy. Further studies are warranted to evaluate for any differences in optimal timing of baseline and follow-up post-therapy PET/CT in patients treated with immunotherapy compared with chemoradiation therapy.

SUMMARY

PET/CT is a valuable tool in the post-therapy follow-up of head and neck cancers. PET/CT is sensitive and specific, can detect recurrences that otherwise may be missed on routine clinical examination or conventional imaging, and also can have an impact on patient management. NCCN guidelines recommend PET/CT be performed within 3 months to 6 months after therapy.

After this baseline scan, however, further routine PET/CT follow-up in asymptomatic patients has unclear benefit, particularly in those with HPV-related disease, which has more favorable prognosis but also tends to recur later in the disease course. Additional post-therapy PET/CT imaging should be individualized to patients based on considerations, such as tumor type, stage, prognostic factors, symptoms, and clinical assessment. Liquid biopsy, such as with circulating or salivary HPV DNA in HPV-related tumors, has emerged as a noninvasive method of detecting disease recurrence and complementing PET/CT follow-up.

CLINICS CARE POINTS

- PET/CT plays an important role in post-therapy follow-up of head and neck cancer patients and is sensitive in detecting recurrence and metastasis.
- Baseline post-therapy PET/CT should be performed within 3 months to 6 months after completion of definitive treatment and no earlier than 12 weeks to reduce false-positive results.
- There is limited benefit of routine follow-up PET/CT in asymptomatic patients with a negative baseline PET/CT at 3 months post-therapy. If follow-up PET/CT is performed, yield may be higher earlier in the post-therapy period, although in the subgroup of HPV-related tumors, recurrences tend to occur later in the disease course.
- Additional post-therapy PET/CT imaging should be individualized to patients based on considerations such as tumor type, stage, prognostic factors, symptoms, and clinical assessment.
- Liquid biopsy with biomarkers, such as circulating or salivary HPV DNA, shows potential for complementing PET/CT in detecting recurrence of HPV-related tumors.

DISCLOSURE

The authors have nothing to disclose.

REFERENCES

1. Siegel RL, Miller KD, Jemal A. Cancer statistics, 2020. CA Cancer J Clin 2020;70(1):7–30.
2. Sung H, Ferlay J, Siegel RL, et al. Global cancer statistics 2020: GLOBOCAN estimates of incidence

and mortality worldwide for 36 cancers in 185 countries. CA Cancer J Clin 2021;71(3):209–49.

3. American cancer Society. Cancer Facts & Figures 2021. American cancer Society. Available at: https://www.cancer.org/content/dam/cancer-org/research/cancer-facts-and-statistics/annual-cancer-facts-and-figures/2021/cancer-facts-and-figures-2021.pdf. Accessed April 30, 2021.

4. National Cancer Institute. Head and neck cancers. National cancer Institute. 2017. Available at: https://www.cancer.gov/types/head-and-neck/head-neck-fact-sheet. Accessed April 30, 2021.

5. Burtness B, Harrington KJ, Greil R, et al. Pembrolizumab alone or with chemotherapy versus cetuximab with chemotherapy for recurrent or metastatic squamous cell carcinoma of the head and neck (KEYNOTE-048): a randomised, open-label, phase 3 study. Lancet 2019;394(10212):1915–28.

6. Goel R, Moore W, Sumer B, et al. Clinical Practice in PET/CT for the management of head and neck squamous cell cancer. AJR Am J Roentgenol 2017; 209(2):289–303.

7. Taghipour M, Sheikhbahaei S, Marashdeh W, et al. Use of 18F-Fludeoxyglucose-Positron emission tomography/computed tomography for patient management and outcome in oropharyngeal squamous cell carcinoma: a review. JAMA Otolaryngol Head Neck Surg 2016;142(1):79–85.

8. Ichimiya Y, Alluri K, Marcus C, et al. Imaging modality utilization trends in patients with stage III-IV oropharyngeal squamous cell carcinoma. Am J Nucl Med Mol Imaging 2015;5(2):154–61.

9. Kim SA, Roh JL, Kim JS, et al. 18)F-FDG PET/CT surveillance for the detection of recurrence in patients with head and neck cancer. Eur J Cancer 2017;72: 62–70.

10. Gupta T, Master Z, Kannan S, et al. Diagnostic performance of post-treatment FDG PET or FDG PET/CT imaging in head and neck cancer: a systematic review and meta-analysis. Eur J Nucl Med Mol Imaging 2011;38(11):2083–95.

11. Taghipour M, Marcus C, Califano J, et al. The value of follow-up FDG-PET/CT in the management and prognosis of patients with HPV-positive oropharyngeal squamous cell carcinoma. J Med Imaging Radiat Oncol 2015;59(6):681–6.

12. Kostakoglu L, Fardanesh R, Posner M, et al. Early detection of recurrent disease by FDG-PET/CT leads to management changes in patients with squamous cell cancer of the head and neck. Oncologist 2013; 18(10):1108–17.

13. Mehanna H, Wong WL, McConkey CC, et al. PET-CT surveillance versus neck dissection in advanced head and neck cancer. N Engl J Med 2016; 374(15):1444–54.

14. National Comprehensive Cancer Network. NCCN clinical Practice guidelines in Oncology: head and neck cancers, version 2.2021. National comprehensive cancer Network. 2021. Available at: https://www.nccn.org/professionals/physician_gls/pdf/head-and-neck.pdf.

15. Denaro N, Merlano MC, Russi EG. Follow-up in head and neck cancer: do more Does it mean do Better? A systematic review and Our Proposal based on Our Experience. Clin Exp Otorhinolaryngol 2016;9(4): 287–97.

16. Sheikhbahaei S, Taghipour M, Ahmad R, et al. Diagnostic Accuracy of follow-up FDG PET or PET/CT in patients with head and neck cancer after definitive treatment: a systematic review and meta-analysis. AJR Am J Roentgenol 2015;205(3):629–39.

17. Gao S, Li S, Yang X, et al. 18FDG PET-CT for distant metastases in patients with recurrent head and neck cancer after definitive treatment. A meta-analysis. Oral Oncol 2014;50(3):163–7.

18. Krabbe CA, Pruim J, Dijkstra PU, et al. 18F-FDG PET as a routine posttreatment surveillance tool in oral and oropharyngeal squamous cell carcinoma: a prospective study. J Nucl Med 2009;50(12): 1940–7.

19. Purohit BS, Ailianou A, Dulguerov N, et al. FDG-PET/CT pitfalls in oncological head and neck imaging. Insights Imaging 2014;5(5):585–602.

20. Porceddu SV, Jarmolowski E, Hicks RJ, et al. Utility of positron emission tomography for the detection of disease in residual neck nodes after (chemo) radiotherapy in head and neck cancer. Head Neck 2005;27(3):175–81.

21. Cheung PK, Chin RY, Eslick GD. Detecting residual/recurrent head neck squamous cell carcinomas using PET or PET/CT: systematic review and meta-analysis. Otolaryngol Head Neck Surg 2016; 154(3):421–32.

22. Van den Wyngaert T, Helsen N, Carp L, et al. Fluorodeoxyglucose-positron emission tomography/computed tomography after Concurrent chemoradiotherapy in locally advanced head-and-neck squamous cell cancer: the ECLYPS study. J Clin Oncol 2017;35(30):3458–64.

23. Kao J, Vu HL, Genden EM, et al. The diagnostic and prognostic utility of positron emission tomography/computed tomography-based follow-up after radiotherapy for head and neck cancer. Cancer 2009; 115(19):4586–94.

24. Beswick DM, Gooding WE, Johnson JT, et al. Temporal patterns of head and neck squamous cell carcinoma recurrence with positron-emission tomography/computed tomography monitoring. Laryngoscope 2012;122(7):1512–7.

25. Boysen ME, Zatterstrom UK, Evensen JF. Self-reported symptoms to monitor recurrent head and neck cancer-analysis of 1,678 cases. Anticancer Res 2016;36(6):2849–54.

26. McDermott M, Hughes M, Rath T, et al. Negative predictive value of surveillance PET/CT in head

and neck squamous cell cancer. AJNR Am J Neuroradiol 2013;34(8):1632–6.

27. Ho AS, Tsao GJ, Chen FW, et al. Impact of positron emission tomography/computed tomography surveillance at 12 and 24 months for detecting head and neck cancer recurrence. Cancer 2013;119(7):1349–56.

28. Mourad M, Jetmore T, Jategaonkar AA, et al. Epidemiological trends of head and neck cancer in the United States: a SEER population study. J Oral Maxillofac Surg 2017;75(12):2562–72.

29. Fakhry C, Westra WH, Li S, et al. Improved survival of patients with human papillomavirus-positive head and neck squamous cell carcinoma in a prospective clinical trial. J Natl Cancer Inst 2008;100(4):261–9.

30. Fakhry C, Zhang Q, Nguyen-Tan PF, et al. Human papillomavirus and overall survival after progression of oropharyngeal squamous cell carcinoma. J Clin Oncol 2014;32(30):3365–73.

31. Subramaniam RM, Alluri KC, Tahari AK, et al. PET/CT imaging and human papilloma virus-positive oropharyngeal squamous cell cancer: evolving clinical imaging paradigm. J Nucl Med 2014;55(3):431–8.

32. Ang KK, Harris J, Wheeler R, et al. Human papillomavirus and survival of patients with oropharyngeal cancer. N Engl J Med 2010;363(1):24–35.

33. Huang SH, Perez-Ordonez B, Weinreb I, et al. Natural course of distant metastases following radiotherapy or chemoradiotherapy in HPV-related oropharyngeal cancer. Oral Oncol 2013;49(1):79–85.

34. Trosman SJ, Koyfman SA, Ward MC, et al. Effect of human papillomavirus on patterns of distant metastatic failure in oropharyngeal squamous cell carcinoma treated with chemoradiotherapy. JAMA Otolaryngol Head Neck Surg 2015;141(5):457–62.

35. Wotman M, Ghaly M, Massaro L, et al. Improving post-CRT neck assessment in patients with HPV-associated OPSCC (Review). Mol Clin Oncol 2020;13(4):24.

36. Corpman DW, Masroor F, Carpenter DM, et al. Post-treatment surveillance PET/CT for HPV-associated oropharyngeal cancer. Head Neck 2019;41(2):456–62.

37. Wang K, Wong TZ, Amdur RJ, et al. Pitfalls of post-treatment PET after de-intensified chemoradiotherapy for HPV-associated oropharynx cancer: Secondary analysis of a phase 2 trial. Oral Oncol 2018;78:108–13.

38. Vainshtein JM, Spector ME, Stenmark MH, et al. Reliability of post-chemoradiotherapy F-18-FDG PET/CT for prediction of locoregional failure in human papillomavirus-associated oropharyngeal cancer. Oral Oncol 2014;50(3):234–9.

39. Helsen N, Van den Wyngaert T, Carp L, et al. FDG-PET/CT for treatment response assessment in head and neck squamous cell carcinoma: a systematic review and meta-analysis of diagnostic performance. Eur J Nucl Med Mol Imaging 2018;45(6):1063–71.

40. Liu HY, Milne R, Lock G, et al. Utility of a repeat PET/CT scan in HPV-associated Oropharyngeal Cancer following incomplete nodal response from (chemo)radiotherapy. Oral Oncol 2019;88:153–9.

41. Su W, Miles BA, Posner M, et al. Surveillance imaging in HPV-related oropharyngeal cancer. Anticancer Res 2018;38(3):1525–9.

42. Spector ME, Farlow JL, Haring CT, et al. The potential for liquid biopsies in head and neck cancer. Discov Med 2018;25(139):251–7.

43. Kong L, Birkeland AC. Liquid biopsies in head and neck cancer: current state and future Challenges. Cancers (Basel) 2021;13(8).

44. Wang Y, Springer S, Mulvey CL, et al. Detection of somatic mutations and HPV in the saliva and plasma of patients with head and neck squamous cell carcinomas. Sci Transl Med 2015;7(293):293ra104.

45. Wuerdemann N, Jain R, Adams A, et al. Cell-free HPV-DNA as a biomarker for oropharyngeal squamous cell carcinoma-A Step towards Personalized medicine? Cancers (Basel) 2020;12(10).

46. Jensen KK, Gronhoj C, Jensen DH, et al. Circulating human papillomavirus DNA as a surveillance tool in head and neck squamous cell carcinoma: a systematic review and meta-analysis. Clin Otolaryngol 2018;43(5):1242–9.

47. Ahn SM, Chan JY, Zhang Z, et al. Saliva and plasma quantitative polymerase chain reaction-based detection and surveillance of human papillomavirus-related head and neck cancer. JAMA Otolaryngol Head Neck Surg 2014;140(9):846–54.

48. Chera BS, Kumar S, Shen C, et al. Plasma circulating tumor HPV DNA for the surveillance of cancer recurrence in HPV-associated oropharyngeal cancer. J Clin Oncol 2020;38(10):1050–8.

49. Tanaka H, Takemoto N, Horie M, et al. Circulating tumor HPV DNA complements PET-CT in guiding management after radiotherapy in HPV-related squamous cell carcinoma of the head and neck. Int J Cancer 2021;148(4):995–1005.

50. Lee JY, Garcia-Murillas I, Cutts RJ, et al. Predicting response to radical (chemo)radiotherapy with circulating HPV DNA in locally advanced head and neck squamous carcinoma. Br J Cancer 2017;117(6):876–83.

51. Rutkowski TW, Mazurek AM, Snietura M, et al. Circulating HPV16 DNA may complement imaging assessment of early treatment efficacy in patients with HPV-positive oropharyngeal cancer. J Transl Med 2020;18(1):167.

52. Veigas F, Mahmoud YD, Merlo J, et al. Immune checkpoints pathways in head and neck squamous cell carcinoma. Cancers (Basel) 2021;13(5).

53. Onesti CE, Freres P, Jerusalem G. Atypical patterns of response to immune checkpoint inhibitors: interpreting pseudoprogression and hyperprogression in decision making for patients' treatment. J Thorac Dis 2019;11(1):35-8.

54. Cohen EEW, Bell RB, Bifulco CB, et al. The Society for Immunotherapy of Cancer consensus statement on immunotherapy for the treatment of squamous cell carcinoma of the head and neck (HNSCC). J Immunother Cancer 2019;7(1):184.

55. Unterrainer M, Ruzicka M, Fabritius MP, et al. PET/CT imaging for tumour response assessment to immunotherapy: current status and future directions. Eur Radiol Exp 2020;4(1):63.

Printed and bound by CPI Group (UK) Ltd, Croydon, CR0 4YY

03/10/2024

01040372-0006